LANDMARKS
IN
MEDICINE

LANDMARKS IN MEDICINE

**Laity Lectures of the
New York Academy of Medicine**

Introduction by
James Alexander Miller, M.D.
President, New York Academy of Medicine

BeardBooks
Washington, DC

v

INTRODUCTION

THE New York Academy of Medicine has long recognized as an obligation the interpretation of the progress of medical knowledge to the public. As long ago as 1886 it was provided in the By-Laws that "The Anniversary Discourse shall be delivered in November and *the public shall be invited to attend."*

In more recent years, appreciating the rapidly growing interest in medical matters, particularly in the field of preventive medicine, and also recognizing the demand for a better mutual understanding between physicians and the community which they serve, the Academy of Medicine extended this service to an annual series of eight lectures.

Other learned societies in various parts of the world have similarly recognized this obligation. Particularly it is interesting to recall the fact that the Royal Institution of England first presented its series of Juvenile Lectures more than a century ago and that Michael Faraday, great and deeply engrossed scientist though he was, found it worth his while to deliver no fewer than nineteen courses of these lectures.

Since those days both science and medicine have progressed with marvelous rapidity and the need, as well as the demand, for a better and wider lay understanding has grown in proportion.

No longer does the physician, seated as a sort of

high priest of medicine, solemnly deliver his pronouncements without explanation or argument, but, rather, he has become the guide and counselor of his patients, sharing as far as possible his knowledge with them and frankly discussing the mutual problems involved.

It is in this spirit of promoting mutual helpfulness and understanding that the Third Series of the New York Academy of Medicine Lectures to the Laity were delivered and are now presented in published form.

They cover a wide field. The reader will be afforded a glimpse of the spirit which guides and inspires the physician's search for new knowledge in Professor Cohn's essay on "The Meaning of Medical Research"; he will find an illuminating essay on "Medicine in the Middle Ages" by Professor James J. Walsh; a concise review of "Medicine and the Progress of Civilization" contributed by Dr. Reginald Burbank; an autobiographic recital of the story of the X-ray by Dr. Lewis Gregory Cole who was a pioneer in the development of this most valuable modern instrument of diagnosis, and also the equally interesting and informing essays of Doctors Packard, Martland, and Pearl.

The New York Academy of Medicine is grateful to these authors for the time, interest and effort they devoted to the preparation and delivery of these lectures, for through them the Academy has again been able to meet one of its important obligations to the community.

JAMES ALEXANDER MILLER, M.D.
President, The New York Academy of Medicine

CONTENTS

I

FROM BARBER-SURGEONS TO SURGEONS

The Evolution of Surgery

BY

FRANCIS R. PACKARD, M.D.
EDITOR OF *Annals of Medical History*

I

FROM BARBER-SURGEONS TO SURGEONS

THE EVOLUTION OF SURGERY AS A PROFESSION

In ancient times among the Greeks and Romans there was no distinction between physicians and surgeons. The greatest of all the Greek writers on medicine, Hippocrates (460-390 B.C.), wrote not only on purely medical matters but also left us some most notable writings on surgical subjects. Hippocrates' work on fractures and dislocations was regarded by Malgaigne, the great French surgeon and medical historian, as one of the best contributions ever made to surgical literature, and many of Hippocrates' clinical case reports are of surgical cases.

Galen (A.D. 130-200) who died at the close of the second century A.D., was the chief authority on what we would now call internal medicine for seventeen centuries, and a great experimental physiologist, but he also practiced surgery, telling us of various operations he performed and that he bought his sutures in a shop on the Via Sacra.

Soranus, somewhat earlier than Galen, was especially famous as an obstetrician and gynecologist, but also distinguished as a surgeon. Later, Oribasius, the physician of the Emperor Julian, the Apostate, Alex-

ander of Tralles, and Paul of Egina, all left contributions to surgery as well as to medicine in their
writings.

It would hardly be worth-while to devote much
consideration to the state of surgery during the centuries designated as the Dark Ages (A.D. 476-1000)
which followed the fall of the Roman Empire. Along
with all other learning and science medical science
sunk to the lowest ebb. Towards the close of this dire
period a special reason arose for the decline of surgery. All learning, including medicine such as it was,
had remained in the bosom of the Church, chiefly
in the monasteries. All physicians, those who practiced medicine, were clerics. But the ecclesiastical
authorities found that the practice of medicine, especially by monks, led to certain abuses. The clerical
or monkish physician frequently sought the fees incident to his practice rather than carry out his less
profitable duties to the Church; the close physical
contact with the bodies of his patients was shocking
to ecclesiastical modesty, and lastly, a priest or monk
should be more concerned with the welfare of the
immortal soul, than with that of the corruptible body.
Therefore in the twelfth and thirteenth centuries
various Councils of the Church issued decrees against
the practice of medicine by churchmen. These decrees were especially directed against any form of surgery, particularly those issued by the Council of
Tours, 1163, and of Le Mans, 1247, wherein the
principal, *ecclesia abhorret a sanguine,* was enunci-
ated with anathemas for those who should violate it.

Internal medicine continued to be practiced by churchmen for some centuries but henceforth the practice of surgery was taboo.

There were, however, some notable exceptions, some clerics who continued to practice not only medicine but surgery. One of these deserves special notice. Guy de Chauliac (1300-1370) although an ecclesiastic, studied anatomy at Bologna and medicine and surgery at Toulouse, Montpellier, and Paris. His *Chirurgia Magna* (1360) went through many editions and was regarded as a standard textbook as late as the seventeenth century. An epitome of it, *Chirurgia parva,* generally known as the *Guidon,* was also very popular. In spite of his fame as a surgeon, Guy was "commensal chaplain" and physician to no less than three popes, Clement V, Innocent VI, and Urban VI, all of whom resided at Avignon during the Great Schism. As Allbutt says, "It is remarkable that around the papal chair the velvet of the hand of the Church was thicker than the iron. In the air of Rome or of Avignon the grim rigor of Paris was marvelously softened."

THE RISE OF THE UNIVERSITIES

The twelfth century was marked by the emergence of the great universities, most of them developing from preëxisting monastic schools. By creating these institutions of higher learning the Church maintained its hold on the intellectual life, just as it already controlled the spiritual life.

The universities gave degrees in medicine of which the recipients were always ecclesiastics. Thus great medical schools arose in the Italian universities of Bologna, Padua, and elsewhere; in France at Paris, Toulouse, and Montpellier; and in England at Oxford. From them were graduated the men who practiced medicine but, though many of these physicians wrote and practised what they called surgery, most of them disdained to do any of the manual work of surgery: bleeding, cupping, and more serious operations such as amputations, the removal of stone in the bladder, trephining, or the reduction of fractures and dislocations. These were left almost entirely in the hands of the laymen, barber-surgeons, or lay brothers in monasteries, or itinerant operators, quacks who wandered about proclaiming their ability as operators. In Italy some of these itinerant, irregular operators acquired great fame such as the Norsini family, who operated for stone in the bladder and hernia, and the Brancas, father and son, who were famous for their skill in restoring noses which had been cut off in fights or as a legal punishment.

THE PROGRESS OF SURGERY IN FRANCE
TO THE TIME OF AMBROISE PARÉ

In the early years of the fourteenth century courses in surgery were given at the University of Paris. Among the teachers were three remarkable men: Lanfranc, an Italian who had been exiled from Milan because of political troubles and whose *Grande*

Chirurgie was a notable contribution to the surgical literature of the time; Jean Pitard, who is revered as the founder of the organization of surgeons known as the Confraternité de Saint-Côme; and Henri de Mondeville, whose treatise on surgery was highly esteemed. These professors had studied at universities and were clerics but did not take orders and they actually practised surgery, operating, dressing wounds, and so on. But shortly after they had passed away we find a very different state of things. Lectures for those who intended to become surgeons continued to be given but no practical surgery was taught and the so-called surgeons of the University of Paris abstained entirely from the actual practice of surgery. Finally in 1350 the Faculty of Medicine passed a decree by which all those who were admitted to its medical courses were required to take an oath never to practise manual surgery.

It may well be asked what were the functions of a surgeon who did not operate, reduce fractures or dislocations, or perform the most usual duties associated with his calling?

In the first place these so-called surgeons associated themselves into an organization or guild, the Confrérie de Saint-Côme, taking for their patron saints, Saint-Côme and St. Damien, those saints being everywhere regarded as the special patrons of the art of surgery. The members of the Confrérie arrogated to themselves the privilege of wearing a long gown, and hence became known as Surgeons of the Long Robe. They were privileged to hang a banner in the

windows of their houses bearing the effigies of their
patron saints with three boxes adorned with golden
fleurs-de-lys at their feet. The Confraternity was supposed to exercise some control over the practice of
surgery in Paris, examining candidates for practice
and granting them licences to do so. From their membership were chosen the sworn surgeons to the king
who served at the prison of the Châtelet. The members of the Confrérie were exempt from duty with
the watch. As far as their practice was concerned,
they were supposed to be called in consultation by the
barber-surgeons or other practitioners of surgery in
all difficult cases. As they would not practice manual
surgery, and as the Faculty of Medicine would not allow them to give medicines internally, their practice
was confined to ordering local applications, ointments,
plasters, lotions, and so forth, and giving learned
advice.

Malgaigne writes with just contempt of these so-
called surgeons and their Confrérie, which later was
transformed into the Collège de Saint-Côme. Its membership was always very limited and it was in constant
hot water between the Faculty of Medicine of the
University of Paris which was continually trying to
keep them down, and the company of the Barber-
Surgeons, whose members really practised surgery
and who constantly sought to encroach on the privileges of the Confrérie. Thus the surgeons tried on
occasions to bring the Barber-Surgeons in subjection
to them by claiming that the latter should be subject
to examination by them before being allowed to prac-

tice surgery. The Barber-Surgeons, supported by the
Faculty of Medicine always succeeded in evading this
claim and asserting their own rights to license barber-
surgeons to practise surgery.

The company or guild of barbers of Paris dates
back to the beginning of the thirteenth century. They
not only cut hair and shaved but also dressed wounds,
bled, cupped, and leeched. Their ensign was the
familiar red and white striped pole with a basin attached to signify that they practiced bleeding. For
many years a triangular fight was maintained. The
surgeons of the Confrérie de Saint-Côme endeav-
oring to subject the barbers to their authority and to
interfere with their practice of surgery and, at the
same time, trying to assert their own privileges against
the Faculty of Medicine, which in its turn lost no
opportunity of asserting its authority over these Surgeons of the Long Robe. Both the Barbers and the
Surgeons of the Long Robe kept appealing in turn
to the Faculty of Medicine to take their part in
these constant bickerings. Finally in 1510 peace was
brought about by a mutual agreement. To the Faculty of Medicine was given authority over both corporations. Both surgeons and barber-surgeons were
required to attend courses given by its teachers, the
barber-surgeons to receive instruction in anatomy and
surgery. Such barbers as desired to practise surgery,
to become barber-surgeons, were required to pass an

examination before the sworn physician and two surgeons of the King at the Châtelet. This agreement
opened the way which later led to barber-surgeons
being admitted to the Confrérie de Saint-Côme and
to Surgeons of the Long Robe becoming doctors-
regent in the faculty. A few years later the vanity of
the Surgeons of the Long Robe was further gratified
by the transformation of their company from the
Confrérie de Saint-Côme into the College of Surgeons
of Paris.

AMBROISE PARÉ

In 1510 there was born in the town of Laval in
Normandy Ambroise Paré, destined to win the well
earned title of the Father of Modern Surgery. There
were several barber-surgeons in his family and after
serving some time probably with a brother who practiced that profession at Vitré, young Paré came to
Paris where he passed some years working in the
Hôtel Dieu. We next find him as an army surgeon in
an expedition into Italy. Although he had not yet
been admitted even to the Barber-Surgeons he went
as surgeon with the soldiers of Marshal de Montejan,
colonel-general of the French infantry. There was no
regular army medical service at this time, command-
ing officers taking with them surgeons as they saw
fit, the surgeon's duty being first to attend his employer and any other officers who needed his services,
and then afterward such soldiers as he could. We cannot follow Paré through his various campaigns of
which he himself when seventy-five years old pub-

lished a charming account in his famous *Apology for His Life and Account of his Journeys in various Places*. Here we are chiefly concerned with his services to the surgical profession. Returning to Paris in 1541 after his first campaign, Paré, at the age of thirty-one, passed his examinations and was admitted to the Community of the Barber-Surgeons. During the rest of his active life Paré served as an army surgeon in many campaigns. In the intervals between them he practised surgery in Paris and wrote many books containing the fruits of his experience. His skill, courage and industry brought him the favorable attention of many powerful nobles and officers. Antoine de Bourbon, King of Navarre, recommended him to King Henry II who made him one of his surgeons, and he subsequently was surgeon to all three of his sons, François II, Charles IX, and Henry III, as well as to Catherine de Medici and many of the nobility.

In 1554 Paré was admitted a member of the Collège de Saint-Côme, thereby becoming a Surgeon of the Long Robe instead of a barber-surgeon. This unprecedented honor was conferred on Paré by the members of the Collège de Saint-Côme in response to a direct mandate from King Henri II. The surgeons were naturally anxious to number among themselves a man of such prominence and weight at Court. According to the regulations of the Collège Paré should have undergone an examination, conducted in Latin, and have written a thesis in the same language. But Paré knew no Latin and there is no record of his having presented a thesis. In short, the surgeons were so eager to have a man of his influence as a member of the Collège that they gladly abrogated their rules in his favor especially when ordered to do so by the King. He was also given his mastership in the Collège without being required to pay the customary fees. Some years later, in 1567, Paré tried to bring all those who should undertake to practise surgery in France under the jurisdiction of the first surgeon to the King, an office then held by himself. Heretofore, the first barber-surgeon to the King had been the ostensible head of not only the barber-surgeons but also the surgeons. Paré petitioned King Charles IX to this effect, but the King referred the matter to the Faculty of Medicine and it was defeated by them. The first barber-surgeon to the King retained the control of all those who practiced surgery in France until Fagon, first surgeon to Louis XIV, finally succeeded in freeing the surgeons from his subjection. Paré had an encounter with the Faculty of Medicine when he published the first collected edition of his works in 1575. It was written in French and dedicated to King Henri III. The Faculty of Medicine formulated a demand that before being put on sale the works of Ambroise Paré, *"homme très impudent et sans aucun savoir,"* should be submitted to them for their approval, and the dean of the Faculty quoted a decree of the *Parlement de Paris* passed in 1535 prohibiting the publication of any book on medicine without permission having been previously obtained from the Faculty of Medicine. Besides which Paré's book contained a section on fevers and much else bearing on medical (non-surgical) topics, and it was written in French because Paré was totally ignorant of Greek and Latin. When the case came up before the *Parlement de Paris* not only did the Faculty of Medicine make their complaint as stated above, but the surgeons of Saint-Côme, probably actuated by jealousy, joined the hue and cry against the author, and the Provost of Paris demanded that the book should be burned because it contained indecencies and things hurtful to morals. Fortunately the book was already on sale and had been widely distributed. The *Parlement de Paris* contented itself with a reaffirmation of the decree of 1535 requiring all medical writings to be submitted to the Faculty of Medicine for its approval before publication, and took no further steps against Paré. This great book marked an epoch in surgery. The very fact that it dealt with medicine as well as surgery was a great step towards bringing about a proper relationship between the two main branches of medicine; and it was written in French and, therefore, could be read by all.

Paré's fame rests on many things besides his services to the Collège de Saint-Côme. I can only mention a few of his most famous achievements:

1. Before his time the opinion prevailed that gunshot wounds were poisoned because of some venomous property in gunpowder. They were treated by pouring boiling oil in the wound. On Paré's first campaign his supply of oil gave out and he had nothing to use on his wounded but a mixture of white of eggs, turpentine and oil of roses. He passed a sleep-

less night wondering in what condition he would find his patients in the morning. When he visited them he found they were all more comfortable and they recovered better than those on whom the boiling oil had been used. Needless to say he never used the latter again.

2. It was customary to stop bleeding after amputation by cauterizing the wound with hot irons, though ligatures were used to stop bleeding in operations for aneurysms, and the like, when vessels were wounded in continuity. Frequently after cauterizing an amputated extremity a slough would form and when it came away the wound would have to be cauterized again to stop the secondary hemorrhage. Paré was the first to use the ligature after amputation.

3. By publishing his works in French, instead of Latin, Paré did a great service to the barber-surgeons who, ignorant of Latin, were unable to avail themselves of any worth-while writings on their work. The anatomical part of his collected works was chiefly a transcript of Vesalius' great book *De Fabrica humani corporis,* but as such it rendered a first-class treatise on anatomy familiar to those who most needed it.

Lastly Paré's personal influence and character had an immense influence in raising the status of the practice of surgery. He had lifted himself from the ranks of the looked-down-upon barber-surgeons to that of the surgeons, and he not only attended many of the great personages of his day in France, but was regarded by them with affection and esteem. The charming style of his writings unconsciously reveal many of his characteristics. His often used phrase *"Je le pensai, Dieu le guarit,"* is known to all, and the notes appended to his case histories *"addresse de l'auteur," "charité de l'auteur,"* and so on, while showing a naïve personal vanity, lend a very human touch.

The status of French surgery in the seventeenth century was greatly improved by a fortunate event which occurred in 1686, when King Louis XIV after many years of suffering from a fistula in ano, finally allowed his surgeon, Charles François Felix, to operate on it. The operation was completely successful and the monarch's gratitude led him to ennoble Felix in addition to giving him a most generous fee. The operation also added greatly to the surgeon's income in a curious way. In their desire to flatter the King courtiers flocked to Felix to get him to perform the operation upon them, in many instances without any necessity for it, and it is said that many who were afraid to face the ordeal pretended to have done so, carrying out the fraud by wearing ostentatiously large dressings about the parts.

Felix was succeeded as royal surgeon by Georges Mareschal and, in 1724, Louis XV at the suggestion of Mareschal and La Peyronnie created five professorships in the Collège de Saint-Côme. This freed the surgeons from the necessity of attending courses in the Faculty of Medicine, to the great indignation of the physicians. The Faculty protested most vigorously but in vain against this removal of the surgeons from their jurisdiction. A few years later, in 1731, Louis XV established the Académie de Chirurgie and, in 1743, the barbers were entirely separated from the surgeons, forbidden to practise any kind of surgery, and it was ordained that, henceforth, no one could get a degree in surgery without having first become a master of arts. Thus the practice of surgery in France was placed on a level with that of medicine.

In 1792, during the Revolution the Académie de Chirurgie, along with all other bodies or institutions possessing special privileges, was abolished. The government of the first French Republic thought to replace trained physicians and surgeons by creating Ecoles de Santé, which were very imperfectly staffed and equipped and turned our so-called Officers de Santé with very inadequate training. When Bonaparte became First Consul he recognized the defects of the system and, in 1804, revived the old system of training and reconstituted the Faculté de Medicine and Académie de Chirurgie.

SURGEONS AND BARBER-SURGEONS IN ENGLAND

Americans sometimes find difficulty in understanding the distinction which is yet observed in England between those members of the medical profession who are known as physicians and practise strictly medicine, and those known as surgeons, who perform operations, dress wounds, and carry out other surgical procedures. The first group, the physicians, possess the degree of M.D. and are always entitled "doctor," whereas those who practise surgery are only designated "mister." [1]

The late Sir Clifford Allbutt [2] tells an amusing story as illustrating the distinction between the practice of medicine and surgery in England. In 1864 a solemn meeting of the staff of the Leeds Infirmary was summoned to discuss whether it was permissible for physicians to use the newly introduced hypodermic needle. Fortunately the question was decided in the affirmative.

During the early years of the fourteenth century there was a barber's guild in London and there was also a distinct class of surgeons but the barbers, as in France, performed certain surgical procedures such as bleeding, dressing wounds and even major operations, amputations, and cutting for stone. That women as well as men practised surgery is evident from a document dated 1389 in which four men are sworn in as "Masters Surgical" before the Mayor and

[1] In this country no such distinction prevails. When the first medical school in this country, that of the College of Philadelphia, was started, in 1765, an attempt was made to bestow the degree of Bachelor of Medicine on those who had studied satisfactorily for two years with the idea that they would return and take further courses to obtain the degree of M.D. The experiment was abandoned after a few years because most of those who had the degree of M.B. were satisfied to start out in practice without seeking further qualifications.

Since that time our medical schools have given uniform courses to all their students, qualifying equally for the practice of either medicine or surgery, and all those who are legally entitled to practise can pursue any branch of the healing art they may see fit.

[2] "The Historical Relations of Medicine and Surgery to the End of the Sixteenth Century," address delivered at the St. Louis Congress in 1904.

Aldermen in their Court at the Guildhall. They were sworn "to practise truly their trade, and to make faithful oversight of others, both men and women, occupied in cures or using the art of surgery." The surgeons seemed to have attempted to exercise some control over the barbers who undertook surgery for, in 1409, the latter petitioned the mayor and aldermen against attempts to control their practise of surgery. Whereupon the mayor and aldermen re-confirmed the barbers' privileges.

In 1415 the mayor and aldermen appointed two masters from among the barbers to oversee the practise of surgery by members of their craft and two other masters to oversee those who confined themselves to barbery.

When Henry V undertook his great campaign in France which culminated in the victory of Agincourt, on October 25, 1415, his expeditionary force consisted of 6,000 men-at-arms and 24,000 infantrymen. He took with him his physician, Nicholas Colnet, and his surgeon, Thomas Morstede. Each of them received twelve pence a day pay, and they each had three archers assigned them as a guard. Morstede also received an allowance of 100 marks each quarter. It is evident that the surgical service to the army was regarded as much more important than the medical, for not alone is Colnet the only physician mentioned to accompany the expedition, but Morstede was ordered to take with him twelve assistant surgeons, each of whom was paid the same pay as an archer, sixpence a day. The King also assigned Morstede "one chariot and two waggons." Morstede was given power to impress surgeons for the service.

In 1435 the surgeons formed themselves into a company, or guild, which though not incorporated, was granted a coat of arms in 1492. Like the Confraternité de Saint-Côme in France, the Guild of Surgeons in England never acquired a very firm footing. As in France they were ground between the physicians and the barber-surgeons and in the end the latter proved too strong for them.

In 1462, Edward IV granted a charter to the Barbers' Company, which gave the Company great power of control over the practice of surgery in London, and which was confirmed by Henry VII in 1497. Finally in 1540 the guild of the surgeons, which had never been incorporated, was united by an act of Parliament with the company of the barbers. Holbein painted a famous picture of Henry VIII granting this charter. He is handing the document to Thomas Vicary, who became the first master of the United Company of Barber-Surgeons. Behind Vicary are kneeling fourteen members of the Barber-Surgeons Company. On the King's right hand are his apothecary and two physicians, the nearest to the King being Sir William Butts who has been immortalized in Shakespeare's *Henry VIII,* for services to Cranmer when the Privy Council attempted to disgrace him.

With the granting of this charter the Company of Surgeons passed out of existence. There was, however, a provision in the Charter that the members of the new United Company who practised surgery could not practise barbery and vice versa no barbery could practise surgery.

Although England in the sixteenth century did not produce an Ambroise Paré, nevertheless, some of the members of the United Company of Barber-Surgeons were men of skill and integrity. Thomas Vicary, to whom Henry VIII is handing the charter in Holbein's famous picture, was the author of *The Englishman's Treasure, With the true Anatomye of Mans Body*, which was the first book on anatomy in the English language.[3]

There were some notable surgeons in London during the reign of Queen Elizabeth: Thomas Gale (1507-86?), John Banister (1540-1604), and William Clowes (1540?-1604), all of whom had served as army surgeons in the field like Ambroise Paré. Thomas Gale served in Henry VIII's army in France in 1544 and was with Philip II's army at the battle of St. Quentin in 1557. He published a book on surgery in 1563 containing a treatise on gunshot wounds in which he states that wounds made with gunpowder are not poisonous and should not be treated with boiling oil or cauteries, but with soothing dressings. The latter years of his life Gale practiced in London.

John Banister served as surgeon with the English expedition to relieve Havre in 1563, and again with the Earl of Leicester's troops in the Low Countries in 1585, after which he practised in London, where

---

[3] It is said that Vicary's book was published in 1548, but the only known edition which now exists was published in 1577, after Vicary's death.

he distinguished himself by his charitable work
among the poor, especially to disabled soldiers.
Though he wrote several books they are chiefly translations or compilations from the works of others. William Clowes was the most notable of these Elizabethan
surgeons. Like Banister he served in the French campaign in 1563, and while doing so he and Banister
began a friendship which was only terminated by
death. After the campaign he settled in London where
he became surgeon to Christ's and St. Bartholomew's
hospitals. He also received the appointment of surgeon to Queen Elizabeth. In 1583 he resigned from
St. Bartholomew's hospital having been "sent for by
letters from Right Honourable and also by her
Majestie's commandment to goe into the Low Countries to attend upon the Right Honourable the Earle
of Leicester, Lord Lieutenant and Captain General of
her Majestie's forces in those countries." Banister also
served in this campaign. In 1588 Clowes was one of
the surgeons in the fleet which fought the Armada.
In 1591 he published his *Proved Practice for all
young Chirurgians* which is full of interesting cases
and observations drawn from his own experience.

SHAKESPEARE'S REFERENCES TO PHYSICIANS AND SURGEONS

There are many references in the plays of Shakespeare to physicians and surgeons. Shakespeare evidently held the physicians in much higher esteem
than the surgeons. There are two physicians that

figure as characters in the plays. The Doctor in *Macbeth* and King Lear's physician are both represented as cultivated men of good judgment and they both manifest their wisdom in the methods they employ in the difficult mental cases of Lady Macbeth and the demented King. In *All's Well That Ends Well* the deceased father of Helena, a physician named Gerard de Narbonne, is spoken of as a man of learning and skill.

Shakespeare evidently did not hold the surgeons of his day in such high esteem. No surgeon figures as a character in the plays, but their services are frequently called for, as, by Cassio when he has been wounded by Iago, and by Duncan when he bids fetch them to dress the wounded sergeant in *Macbeth*.

In *Troilus and Cressida* there is a pun on the then popular surgical practice of keeping wounds open by a "tent," a piece of cloth or gauze inserted into the wound. Apropos of Achilles sulking in his tent Patroclus demands;

Who keeps the tent now?

To which filthy but witty Thersites replies:

The surgeon's box, or the patient's wound.

But in one instance in which the services of a surgeon are required he is represented as in a sad condition.

In *Twelfth Night* Sir Andrew Aguecheek calls for a surgeon after he and Sir Toby Belch have been wounded by Viola. Sir Toby demands of the Clown:

> Sot, didst see Dick surgeon . . . ?

to which the Clown replies:

> O! he's drunk, Sir Toby, an hour agone. His
> eyes were set at eight i' the morning.

The irate Sir Toby says:

> Then he's a rogue, and a passy measures pavin,

adding virtuously:

> I hate a drunken rogue.[4]

During the seventeenth century there were two surgeons who did much to elevate the status of the profession and pave the way for the separation of the surgeons from the barbers.

John Woodall (1556-1643) began his professional career as a surgeon with Lord Willoughby's regiment in 1591. Woodall passed eight years in Germany and acquired such knowledge of German that he was chosen to act as interpreter to an embassy sent to that country by Queen Elizabeth. He also traveled in France and Poland. Returning to England he was admitted to the Barber-Surgeons Company, of which he subsequently became Master. As his services were still valued in diplomatic circles he accompanied an embassy which James I sent to Poland. Woodall was elected surgeon to St. Bartholomew's Hospital in 1616 where he was a colleague of William Harvey of whom he writes with great esteem. In 1612 he was appointed as the first surgeon-general of the East India Com-

4 *Twelfth Night,* V, 1, 202.

pany, and he was much interested in the affairs of the Virginia Company. But Woodall should be especially noted because he was the first medical writer to direct attention to the value of lime juice in the prevention and treatment of scurvy on ships. In his *The Surgeon's Mate,* which he published in 1617 as a handbook for the use of the surgeons in the employ of the East India Company, he says that "the juice of lemon is a precious medicine." If lemon juice is not procurable Woodall says that the juice of limes, oranges, or citrons, or the pulp of tamarinds, may be used as substitutes. The famous old sea-dog Hawkins had previously used lemon juice for scurvy and proclaimed its value, But Woodall is the first medical authority for its use.

Richard Wiseman (1622?-76) is entitled to be called the English Paré, so closely does his career resemble that of the great Frenchman. After serving his apprenticeship to a barber-surgeon, Wiseman served for some years as a surgeon in the Dutch Navy, in which capacity he saw very active service. In 1643 he joined the royalist army in the west of England, and became attached to the person of Prince Charles, whom he accompanied to France, Holland and Scotland. He was taken prisoner at the battle of Worcester in 1651. Wiseman seems to have been treated with leniency because he was liberated after some weeks when he settled in London to practise. But his restlessness soon led him to a more exciting life. He entered the Spanish service in which he served for three years, part of the time at Dunkirk and some of it in the tropics. In 1660 when Charles II returned, Wiseman was back in London and in the following year he was appointed surgeon to the King, and some years later, sergeant and principal surgeon to him. Wiseman wrote several books of which the most important was *Severall Chirurgical Treatises* (1676). This book is full of reports of cases, accompanied by anecdotes and observations written in racy Elizabethan English. As a good Royalist Wiseman believed firmly in the efficacy of the Royal Touch in the cure of scrofula. As surgeon to the King he witnessed the performance on many occasions.

As showing the high plane on which the United Company wished to conduct their anatomical teaching, in 1548 shortly after their incorporation, they chose as their Reader, or Lecturer, on anatomy, the physician, Dr. John Caius, who had studied at Padua and was a most erudite Greek scholar. He published notable editions of Galen and was the founder of Gonville and Caius College, Cambridge. The custom of choosing a physician, therefore a scholar, to read their lectures on anatomy was continued until the United Company was dissolved in 1745.

It should be recalled that in 1518 Henry VIII had given a charter to the Royal College of Physicians. Thus there were after 1540 two chartered organizations, the physicians and the barber-surgeons, dividing the practice of medicine and surgery in London.

The members of the College of Physicians held themselves very much above their humbler brethren, the Barber-Surgeons, and this arrogant aloofness continued for many generations. Charles II emphasized the pride of the physicians when he ordained, in 1674, that no person should be admitted as a Fellow who had not graduated from Oxford or Cambridge.

As I have said, a distinction was made between those members of the United Company of Barber-Surgeons who practised solely "barbery" and those who practised surgery. Those who practised barbery placed as a symbol in front of their shops the red and white poles with a basin on the top signifying that they could practise bleeding. A very important provision in the charter of the Company was that it each year was allotted "for anatomies" the bodies of four felons who had been duly convicted and executed. These bodies were to be dissected in the hall of the Company, the dissections being presided over by two masters and two stewards chosen annually among the members of the Company.

A rule was passed by the Company forbidding any members of the Company from making "Private anathomies" or dissections elsewhere than in the Hall of the Company. This rule was probably passed because of the difficulty experienced in procuring bodies for dissection except those of the four felons above mentioned, but it wrought great harm to the study of anatomy, because it prevented teachers of anatomy who had private classes or schools from giving practical instruction in the subject on the human body to their pupils. The rule was frequently violated. In 1714 William Cheselden was called to account by the United Company of Barber-Surgeons, being accused of having frequently procured the bodies of executed criminals and dissected them at his house, "and that at time when lectures and dissections were proceeding at the Hall, whereby the attendance at the Hall was diminished, and moreover contrary to the express laws of the Company." Cheselden escaped punishment by promising never to offend again.

In addition to the masters and stewards at a public anatomy there was also a Reader, who for many years was a physician. The term "Public anatomy" was applied to those dissections which were performed on the bodies of criminals allotted to the Company by law, all other dissections being known as "private." The public anatomies were very formal occasions. Pepys has left an account of one which he attended on February 27, 1662/3. He and Commissioner Pett went to the Barber-Surgeons' Hall about eleven o'clock in the morning,

where we were led into the Theater: and by and by comes the Reader Dr. Tearne, with the Master and Company, in a very handsome manner: and all being setled, he begun his lecture; and his discourse being ended, we had a fine dinner and good learned company, many Doctors of Physique, and we used with great respect. Among other observables we drunk the King's health out of a gilt cup given by King Henry VIII to this Company, with bells hanging at it, which every man is to ring by shaking after he hath drunk up the whole cup.

Pepys also speaks with admiration of Holbein's great picture of Henry VIII bestowing the charter in 1540. A few years later Pepys went again to the Hall to see the picture, "thinking to have bought it by the help of Mr. Pierce for a little money: I did think to give £200 for it, it being said to be worth £1,000," adding, "but it is so spoiled that I have no mind to it, and it is not a pleasant though a good picture."

Besides the physicians and the barber-surgeons there arose a third class of legally recognized practitioners of medicine in England. In 1606 the apothecaries were incorporated into a company, the members of which a few years later (1617) were granted a new charter as the Apothecaries of the City of London by which they acquired the right not only to compound and sell drugs, but also to prescribe them, hence to practice medicine. Although they chiefly ran counter to the physicians they also did considerable minor surgery, cupping, leeching, and dressing wounds, and midwifery.

In 1815 the Apothecaries Society was given greatly increased powers by an act of Parliament creating from its members a licensing board which had power to grant the right to practise to those who had done certain work in hospitals and attended courses of lectures provided for them.

You may recall Thackeray's pen picture of Pendennis' father, who was one of this class:

Early in the regency of George, the Magnificent, there lived in a small town in the West of England, called Clavering, a gentleman whose name was Pendennis.

There were those alive who remembered having seen his name painted on a board which was surmounted by a gilt pestle and mortar over the door of a very humble little shop in the city of Bath, where Mr. Pendennis exercised the profession of apothecary and surgeon, and where he not only attended gentlemen in their sick-rooms, and ladies at the most interesting periods of their lives, but would condescend to sell a brown paper plaster to a farmer's wife across the counter, or to vend tooth brushes, hair powder, and London perfumery.

This threefold division of practice among the physicians, surgeons, and apothecaries still continues in England. Since 1886 candidates to practice medicine or surgery are required to pass a conjoint examination held by the Royal College of Physicians of London and the Royal College of Surgeons of England in the subjects of medicine, surgery, and obstetrics, successful candidates receiving a license from the College of Physicians and the diploma of membership in the College of Surgeons. The right of the Apothecaries to grant licentiates the privilege to prescribe or practice is also recognized.

Towards the close of the seventeenth century the surgeons manifested the desire to free themselves from their union with the barbers and in 1745 the separation was finally effected, chiefly through the efforts and influence of two men, John Ranby and William Cheselden.

John Ranby (1703-74) was admitted to the United Company of Barber-Surgeons in 1722. Several years later he became a Fellow of the Royal Society. He was appointed surgeon-in-ordinary to King George II in 1730 and then sergeant-surgeon in which capacity he accompanied his sovereign at the battle of Dettingen, in 1743, that being the last occasion on which a sovereign of England actually accompanied his troops on a campaign, if we except the presence of King George V in the field during the World War, and Ranby was the last sergeant-surgeon to fill the special duties of that position by serving with his king on a field of battle. Ranby's services were not required by the King but he dressed a wound in the leg of the King's son, the Duke of Cumberland. Ranby published a little book entitled *The Method of Treating Gunshot Wounds,* London, 1744, which contains an account of some of his experiences during the campaign in Germany. When the subject of separating the surgeons from the barbers was under consideration in Parliament, Ranby exerted all his great influence in high places to bring it about. After it was accomplished his services were recognized by his election as the first Master of the newly formed Corporation of Surgeons, Joseph Sandford being elected Senior Warden, and William Cheselden Junior Warden.

Ranby presented the Corporation with a silver cup which is still a cherished possession of the Royal College of Surgeons of England. Ranby is said by some of his contemporaries to have been vain and arrogant, but Fielding in *Tom Jones* introduces him as attending with skill and kindness to the injuries received by the "Old Man of the Hill," saying, "He had, moreover, many good qualities, and was a very generous good-natured man, and ready to do any service to his fellow-creatures." Queen Caroline, upon whom he operated unsuccessfully for a strangulated umbilical rupture, called him "a blockhead."

The other man who did most service in bringing about the separation of the surgeons from the barbers was William Cheselden (1688-1752) whose influence was due not to social prestige or position, for he was in disfavor at Court, but to his great contributions to surgical science and his professional standing. Cheselden studied surgery under William Cowper, the most distinguished surgeon of his day, and James Ferne, the best lithotomist in London. At the early age of twenty-four he became a Fellow of the Royal Society because of his descriptions of some archæological remains which were dug up in an old Roman camp near St. Albans.

Cheselden gave private courses on anatomy and published a treatise on that subject which went through many editions. His greatest contribution to scientific literature, *Osteographia, or the Anatomy of the Bones,* was a beautifully illustrated folio volume, dealing not only with the bones of the human body but also with those of many animals, thus constituting it one of the first, well illustrated books on comparative anatomy. There is much humor as well as taste in the arrangement of the illustrations. Thus the skeleton of the cat is shown in an attitude of alarm, with raised back and tail facing the skeleton of a dog. A heron's skeleton is depicted with that of a fish in its bill, and the skeleton of a crocodile is winding its way with a pyramid in the background.

As an operator Cheselden was chiefly renowned for his skill in removing stones from the bladder, and in operations on the eye. In the days before the discovery of anæsthesia rapidity in the performance of an operation was a great factor in the success of a surgeon. A French surgeon recorded that he had seen Cheselden remove a stone from a bladder in fifty-four seconds and that he rarely took more than a few minutes for the operation. In 1728 Cheselden published in the *Philosophical Transactions* of the Royal Society the report of a case which caused a great sensation. He had operated successfully on a boy of thirteen for congenital cataract, and he gave a vivid account of the patient's experience and sensations when he was able to see for the first time. In the same volume Cheselden described the operation of iridectomy, or forming an artificial pupil by making an incision in the iris.

Cheselden was appointed surgeon to the Queen in 1729, but not long after lost his favor at Court because he had requested that he should be allowed to perforate the ear-drum of a deaf criminal who had been sentenced to be hanged, in order that he might study the effect of the operation on the hearing. The man was to be pardoned if he consented to the operation. Cheselden says that the man was taken ill and the operation had to be deferred "during which time there was so great a clamor raised against it, that it was afterwards thought fit to forbid it." As a token of his loss of royal favor Cheselden was not summoned to attend Queen Caroline in her last illness in 1737. The Queen died of a strangulated umbilical hernia, and her life might possibly have been saved by skilful surgical intervention.

Cheselden was a cultivated man, with literary and artistic tastes. He assisted the artist who made the drawings for his *Osteographia* and is said to have drawn the plans for the old bridge over the Thames at Putney and for the Surgeon's Hall in Monkwell Street. He attended Sir Isaac Newton and was a close friend of Sir Hans Sloane. He was also the friend and physician of the poet Pope, who wrote:

> I'll do what Mead and Cheselden advise
> To keep these limbs and to preserve these eyes.

One of the most beneficial effects which followed the separation of the surgeons from the barbers was a great improvement in the methods of teaching anatomy. Owing to the rule of the United Company which practically inhibited teachers of anatomy from using dead bodies for dissection purposes outside of the Hall of the Company, the subject had to be taught chiefly by pictures, charts, wax or plaster models, and injected preparations, all very poor substitutes for actual dissection. The new Surgeons' Company had no such regulation. It was the absence of this hampering which enabled William Hunter to open his anatomical school in London in 1746, one year after the separation, with the announcement that anatomy would be taught after "the French way," the pupils being furnished with human bodies which they could actually dissect. Within a few years many other anatomy schools were established with equal facilities and for many years London was a great center for anatomical teaching. The demand for bodies became so great that a special class of purveyors of dead bodies arose, who got their supplies by robbing graves and were popularly known as "resurrectionists." The anatomists gave large prices for corpses, especially if the body were fresh and in good condition, and the business was so profitable and those who followed it so disreputable that some of them began committing murder to augment their supply. In London two men, Bishop and Williams, were convicted and executed for the murder of a young Italian; but the most sensational developments occurred in Edinburgh where two wretches, Burke and Hare, murdered sixteen or more people before they were caught. These crimes aroused public opinion. Mobs attacked the anatomical school of Robert Knox, the Edinburgh anatomist to whom Burke and Hare had sold most of their victims, and similar attacks were made on anatomical schools elsewhere. Parliament took up the matter and, in 1832, passed an Anatomy Act, which legally assured a sufficient supply of bodies to meet the needs of the anatomy teachers throughout the United Kingdom.

When the surgeons separated from the barbers they had to surrender to the latter the Hall, in which the United Company had met, with the library, plate, and furniture within it. For a while the new Corporation of Surgeons met in the Hall of the Stationers' Company, but they soon built a house of their own in the Old Bailey, conveniently near to the place of execution at Newgate, whence they got their lawfully allotted supply of felons' bodies.

In 1796 the Corporation lost its legal right to exist in a curious way. By its Act of Incorporation its governing body, the Court of Assistants, was to consist of a master, or chief governor, and two governors, or wardens, with other members, of whom it was enacted that the master and one governor, together with one or two members, should form a court for the despatch of business. In 1796 a court was held at which the Master, William Cooper, and seventeen members were present, but no governor, one of the two governors having died, and the other being bedridden. The members, in spite of this, held their court, and by this illegal action automatically destroyed their existence.

The members hastened to get a new act of incorporation, but met with many vexations and delays. Finally in 1800 George III reëstablished the Corporation as the Royal College of Surgeons of London. As such it continued until 1843 when a new charter was obtained from Queen Victoria changing its name to the Royal College of Surgeons of England. This charter also created two classes in the membership, fellows and members. Those who received a license from it to practice were known as licentiates and were eligible subsequently to election to membership under certain conditions.

II

THE MEANING OF MEDICAL RESEARCH

BY

ALFRED E. COHN, M.D.

MEMBER OF THE ROCKEFELLER INSTITUTE FOR MEDICAL RESEARCH,
NEW YORK

II

THE MEANING OF MEDICAL RESEARCH

I COULD enliven this report by a description of discoveries, dramatic and exciting perhaps; of new diseases or of the mechanisms underlying diseases already identified; of new drugs which cure, like sulphanilamide; or of new operations which relieve or prevent devastating conditions, as for example the great new insights which have resulted from studying the pituitary gland seriously. The investigation of this organ by Cushing who gave the forward movement a great impetus, and by many other very capable and ingenious investigators; has resulted in the description of new ailments, has given point to the attempt to understand the interrelations of fluids and tissues and organs, in ways and to extents not dreamed of ten years ago; has made available agents of real power in adjusting defaulting or erring mechanisms. Or in a sense less pathological and more physiological, I might discuss how great has been the increase in knowledge of the behavior of such important tissues as muscle and nerve. To report on any one of these topics adequately would take too long. There are ample provisions, however, for spreading that sort of information. My task is both simpler and more complicated—to discuss what research in medicine "means," what its nature is and what its purposes. And I take that to include an inquiry into its position in the complicated matrix of our social structure.

The ultimate meaning or purpose of medical research is to rid men of diseases, to protect them from maladies with which they are threatened, to relieve them of discomforts once they are established. There are many diseases, differing in the degree of dangerousness, differing in nature, differing in geographic distribution. There are pathological states to the existence of which we are sensitive—others which, for various reasons, we ignore. Then there is the character of education, having its sources and momentum in the contemporary scene, which makes men fit to undertake chiefly what is comprehensible in that scene. Researches are delayed because points of importance are missed, scholars being unprepared to comprehend them and to seize their opportunities. Researches are sometimes hurried, wasteful, and erroneous, because the idea is entertained that current equipment is adequate to deal with particular problems. The question of public versus private scholarship is important—less important now when the whole situation of research is better understood, and when private scholarship is recognized as being less private than formerly. Private refers both to financial resources sufficient to free scholars from the restrictions imposed upon the use of public funds; and to intellectual latitude which makes room for personal vagary, for unorthodoxy, which may not be tolerated even in an academic environment. But greater in importance than either, because essential, is the pervasiveness of current belief and opinion, current social need, the implications in the current social scene, which tend to influence or, perhaps better, which do not permit us to escape current intellectual compulsions. These are aspects of the intellectual life of which Hessen and his followers have made us aware.[1]

The meaning of medical research must regard these various social and personal aspects. It must regard also the nexus which exists between medical and other sciences. It must make an effort to understand likenesses and differences which characterize medicine in relation to those other sciences. It must analyze the situations, diseases, and social pressures, to which energy is devoted and must describe the means, in men and facilities, which are available for carrying them out.

---

[1] It would be interesting and important to study the nature of social pressure, using this term in its widest sense, in the province of diseases. It is a point of view not strange to historians and students of social phenomena, but one not yet much employed in medical thinking. The illustrations in this essay have been drawn chiefly from communicable diseases and from a few other maladies differently grouped. But the relations exhibited by the development of knowledge of nutrition, or of understanding chemical processes on which nutrition depends, of agricultural growth, of social change in which the demands on the food supply of the less favored receive more sympathetic recognition—all these are matters which lie for analysis at the door of the critic. Here, as elsewhere, these and other factors require study in a complete account of the processes at work in a community.

I propose to discuss first, of *what* we study; second, of *how* we study it; third, of *who* does the studying; and finally, in the course of this discussion, *for what reason* does the study take place.

When these far-reaching issues and conceptions are being canvassed there must first be described certain situations which the world of diseases presents to investigators. It has already been suggested that these vary with time and place. We do not study those diseases which do not exist—or which exist elsewhere, or which exist no longer. The impulse to study a given disease or a given hygienic circumstance results from the danger or the damage which its presence causes. Epidemics of diseases like the black death, or of poliomyelitis, or of influenza, or of cholera, can scarcely or safely be ignored. But not many of the resources of this community are devoted to yellow fever, or kala-azar, or African sleeping sickness. If these diseases were, by their maritime introduction, to threaten the local population, a study of them would be inescapable. They are studied though for several reasons; a general philanthropic motive, because, as in the opinion of Dr. Albert Schweitzer, restitution should be made by a people for the injury done another, because to study them is imperative to preserve health along international trade routes. Pressure of some sort is usually experienced or is exercised when a study is undertaken.

Of the diseases which we do study, there are several kinds. It is of very great importance to understand that diseases cannot, all of them, be regarded as forming a system. They can be grouped, as indeed they are, to form several systems. The various systems have, superficially at least, little in common except that they transform the individuals whom they afflict.[2] Each group, on the other hand, exhibits traits which leave no, or little, doubt as to the relatedness of the members.

The center of gravity of interest in diseases has long, roughly for two generations, lain in *infectious* and *epidemic diseases*. To understand them and to cure them, the sciences which needed to be and which were and are actively cultivated, are bacteriology and parasitology—these two in some respects similar. More recently diseases resulting from viruses, agents of far smaller dimensions than bacteria, have been added to the list. These diseases all depend on the invasion of animal and plant organisms by these agents. Parallel with bacteriology and parasitology, sciences, roughly grouped as immunological, have been developed, in which there have been studied the reactions, that is to say, the behavior of the hosts, plants and animals, which the infectious agents invade. Studies of immunity have gone farther, though, than the study of individual hosts when under attack. A science of epidemiology has grown alongside the other sciences in order to study the conditions in

---

[2] A disease is not an "entity"—it is a transformed organism. The organism is conditioned for exhibiting disease by processes which dispose it to this exhibition. The preparation may be constitutional or psychological or local—but the transformed organism is transformed, not solely by what is called an invader.

which societies of men, animals, and plants, chance to become prepared for invasion by infecting agents. These include external factors—climate, race, season, sunlight; and internal factors—the blood, the plasma, certain organs and tissues, heredity. To cope with these invasions, efforts in various directions have sedulously been made—with sera, which utilize the forces animal bodies themselves prepare for their protection; with chemicals, like salvarsan, like optochin, like arsphenamine, sulphanilamide—all synthetized with the utmost chemical skill; with natural pharmacal agents, chaulmoogra oil, quinine, salicylates. These are, in a sense, beginnings, the success of which points to the fact that the way of thinking about such problems as they represent, is sound and therefore encouraging. Much more may be expected from such efforts. Indeed, not more than auspicious beginnings have been made.

A point of importance, later to be referred to, is that the successes, still in many instances not more than partial, have been attained by delving below the surface of naturally existing phenomena, of appearances, to learn on what these diseases depend. The rewarding results have been that bacteria have been found, and protozoa and viruses. With this kind of knowledge as a background, substances of many sorts were, and are, being sought to oppose the action of the invaders. Here are the rudiments of analytical procedures. They represent something new in the study of diseases. Compared to the amount of energy which has been expended the success so far achieved has, quite obviously, been extraordinary.

Infectious or contagious or epidemic diseases have often been characterized as acute. Acute means two things—that individuals are seized suddenly with disability, a matter of hours or minutes; and also that their duration is usually brief, though there are numerous exceptions, as tuberculosis, syphilis, and leprosy.

But there are long drawn out ailments, often called *chronic,* which fall into two great groups. Certain ones occur at all ages, like pernicious anæmia or diabetes mellitus. But there are others which befall older persons exclusively. I designate these, "ailments" and not "diseases," nor yet degenerative—two words often applied to them which I prefer not to use—for reasons which I hope later to develop.

To distinguish diseases merely according to their duration is a crude conception. But to do so has a use, for the time being. Chronic has usually been intended to signify long drawn out. Roughly, chronic and long drawn out mean the same thing. From the point of view of patients and their families, duration is important; and from that of administrators concerned with the public health, the distinction is essential. Actually what is involved is the rate at which the processes in different maladies advance. Chronic diseases or long drawn out maladies include a wide range of complaints. Their duration is to be estimated, naturally, from their beginning to their termination, uninfluenced, when such examples are available, by treatment. The group is diverse; there are, for example, the diseases of the blood-forming organs—pernicious anemia, leucemia, thrombopenia; there is cancer; there is tuberculosis; there are the deformities of the joints; there are cardiac and arterial derangements; there are the defects which result from insufficience or malfunction of the glands of internal secretion, the hormones in short; there are diseases of the nervous system. It has been customary to divide diseases into three, or perhaps better two, main groups as I am doing; bacteriological and physiological both, but the latter especially employing physical and chemical technics. Chronic diseases fall into each of them. These categories require in certain instances to be stretched fairly wide, in order to include all the varieties. But they will serve for this discussion, especially if in studying bacterial diseases, the behavior of the host, immunology, is included; and if in the physiological ones, anatomical defects and malformations.

It is sufficient, I think, to suggest that medicine deals with many kinds of conditions and that they fall roughly into the categories that have been indicated. Of chief moment is that the classification, though rough, suffices to indicate that well characterized groups can be recognized and that through this possibility study is facilitated, perhaps made possible.

Now it is generally understood and, indeed, it must be obvious, that when a malady or any other natural phenomenon begins to be *analyzed* (analysis being the method essential to experimental research) very soon a level of organization is reached, less complex than the native state of a whole plant or animal, the study of which requires recourse to a chemical laboratory. This is due to the fact that biological mechanisms, when the attempt is made to view them more simply, break down promptly to chemical processes. In physiological diseases, especially those of the heart and arteries, in parallel fashion, a stage is reached when mechanical and physical appliances are needed to help in understanding what is going on. To turn to chemistry, to mechanics, to physics, is to turn not so much to fundamental things, as to machinery which underlies and which determines more complex, directly observable behaviors. These disciplines—physics, chemistry, immunology—constitute the technics which are used to analyze, to reduce to simpler, more easily understandable mechanisms, the surface appearance of maladies. The fact that this is the situation in research in diseases constitutes a dilemma. To this problem it will be necessary to return.

I have referred to *two kinds of chonic diseases*—one which can occur at any age and one which is characteristic of the aged. Those diseases characteristic of the aged require especial description because, though they are not new, they are beginning to take on new significance. We grow older, all of us. As is well known, in the course of doing so we fall subject predominantly to several distinct kinds of disabilities. I pass over cancer; its nature and its ravages are in every one's mind. But what happens to the heart, the arteries, and the kidneys, has been less clearly appreciated. I do not wish to discuss all the possibilities, all the theories. One theory ought, I think, to be more fully described. In the sense that everybody ages, aging has come to be looked upon as a natural phenomenon—natural as differing from accident or from chance. Since every one ages, aging is anticipated and the separate phenomena of aging are looked upon as predictable. This has been a subject of very active research in recent years. And the objectives in such researches have been twofold: first, to ascertain as precisely as possible a picture of what actually takes place and second, to discover what mechanisms are at work to bring about such results. I single out the arteries for more detailed description. That the arteries change is now universally known, especially the great artery of the body, the aorta. What is less well known is that the smaller ones do also. Arteries which have come in for marked attention in recent years are those of the heart, the coronary arteries. The walls of arteries may be thought of as having layers or coats. In the coronary arteries, for example, the first detectable changes take place in the innermost layer; its elastic membrane splits in two and does so rather early in life, in the twenties. From then on, more and more changes take place. At fifty or sixty these changes are advanced and have been termed arterio-sclerosis. To one familiar with the succession of these appearances, it is possible to tell their age, within a few years. Being able to do this is good evidence that there is nothing haphazard about the process. How are these systematic changes brought about? And how, assuming that they develop systematically, can they be prevented or delayed? To answer these questions, guesses have been ventured since very early times and to explain them, serious, far-reaching researches have been undertaken. But so far there are no answers satisfactory to many scientists. Meanwhile the quest goes on with intensifying earnestness. The problem, as I shall show presently, is urgent. What is true of the arteries of the heart is true of those of the brain. About other organs less is known. Progressive alterations, appropriate to each organ and tissue, go on throughout the body— beside the heart muscle, in the kidneys, in the liver —everywhere in short.

But changes in structure do not alone exhibit progressive alteration. Comparable ones can be observed also in the functioning of the body. The slow and gradual rise with age which the blood pressures exhibit are well known. Another striking one has recently been found in the nutrition of the body. Here, it appears that ptyalin, the starch-splitting ferment of the saliva, decreases between twenty-five and eighty-one (these are averages) to one thirty-fourth, necessitating, it seems probable, a very striking readjustment in digestion and food requirements in the aged. More intimate still are changes in behavior of the muscle fibers of the heart. It has been shown in dogs, for example, that as the animals grow older, the ability of this tissue to utilize oxygen diminishes significantly. Finally, as in changes in structure and in function, so also, it appears, can changes in psychological performance be detected. Interest in this phase of growth has begun more recently, so that it would be rash to accept the results of preliminary studies. There can be little doubt though that this is a fruitful field for further investigation.[3]

Many regard it as an idle question, but it is one which should be put, nevertheless—are processes so universal as those identified with aging, to be classed with diseases? Diseases are not constant; they wax and wane; new ones occur; old ones vanish; they are unlooked for; they are recovered from. Of the changes which accompany aging, none of these characteristics can be predicated. It seems better to weigh the question of the nature of this process of aging a while longer, before coming to a decision on its nature. Two ways of thinking are possible—that aging is an accident which can be prevented; or that it is not an accident and that as the body increases in bulk, and by so doing is said to grow, parallel changes are taking place within the body, in its most intimate recesses, which accompany that growth, and which themselves may be regarded as taking part in, and perhaps constituting, the phenomena of growth. In this sense the body grows continuously, changes,

[3] This reference to psychological matters is brief because I am depending on other phases of this problem for illustration. But the place in human nature and in diseases which psychological deviations occupy can scarcely be overemphasized. I am at one with those who wish to understand organisms as wholes and to return from the wilderness into which the requirements of thought in the seventeenth century naturally led us.

called differentiation, taking place in all its parts, the form of change passing from stage to stage without break until the final dissolution. This view urges that there is only one forward moving change—not, first growth and then degeneration, but continuous progressive differentiation. And growth so understood is not an accident, it is not degeneration, and it is not disease.

These old ailments present a new challenge. To care for them is becoming a great burden, financially. Can anything be done to relieve the strain? Medical research, not yet very consciously, is struggling with the question. It has no settled answer. When such questions were first raised fifteen years ago, we were not yet ready to weigh them. Now the response may become, is indeed becoming, more intelligent. The old hospitals built for infectious diseases will no longer serve. In part they are improperly constructed for these purposes. And from the point of view of research, the new situation calls for new orientation. It is still inescapable that research in infectious diseases continue here and elsewhere. Here because there is still tuberculosis, syphilis, poliomyelitis and other infections of the nervous system, rheumatic fever, and influenza; elsewhere, in the tropics, because of diseases indigenous there, but perhaps transplantable here. But since the dawn of that era in which we have spent our lives, the emphasis has been almost exclusively on diseases of this kind. It would be incorrect to say that diseases longer drawn out at older ages had been neglected, cancer, for example, or cardiac diseases. But it is certain that in comparison with infectious diseases, they have been much less cared for and studied. The great desideratum now, is to turn increasing attention to these conditions. If they were better understood, it might become possible to manage them better. If they were better treated, expensive care in homes and in institutions might be less necessary; if they were less expensively treated, the burden of taxation might diminish. The net result would accrue vastly to the sufferers themselves in increased health, in greater freedom spent outside of institutions, in greater economic self-sufficiency. Psychologically, the lives of older men and women might be re-made if we learned how to make them self-sufficient to a degree impossible now, through a new orientation to employment, utilizing opportunities for activity appropriate to the aged. Embedded in the matrix of our society, no better fate is provided for them or envisaged than progressive deterioration.

I have been discussing *what* we study. I come now to *how* we do so. After long reflection and practical experience, there has come to be general comprehension of the purposes and methods of the sciences in general. By the same token, a similar statement can be made of medical science. But in some subtle way, there is tacit agreement that the two are in essence, somehow different. Whether they are, depends I think upon the aspect from which this judgment is made. They do not differ, there would be general agreement in attitude to natural phenomena; nor do they differ in the seriousness with which the problems of diseases are studied; nor do they differ in the methods which both, or all, use. To recognize and to point out differences is not invidious; no more is intended than to understand a complicated situation.

Two suggest themselves—first, one having to do with the nature of the subject matter; and second, one having to do with the circumstances conditioning the activities of students of diseases. The former difference, in subject matter has, I venture to believe, a certain validity; [4] the second, I think, not. To begin with, though it is not my intention to become involved merely in words, it is well to make clear the meaning I ascribe to certain terms.

Science, very briefly, is a way of looking at nature, in so far as that is possible, exactly. Two aspects are involved—the natural phenomena themselves, and a way of looking.

Research is procedure. Research represents the effort men make to increase their comprehension. To discover what is true about anything is an arduous undertaking because, at the outset, so many things

[4] It is perhaps a superficial experience but one to which large numbers of persons are sensitive, that in a very general sense diseases are ugly, repellant, offensive. These are not qualities which characterize phenomena studied in other sciences. The reverse may, and often is, true. It is, of course, a fact that to many men, perhaps especially to physicians, this aspect of diseases is without meaning. It may be that to them the very fact of ugliness has the value of attractiveness. Nor need this be regarded as odd. The last word on the subject of ugliness has not been uttered, in sight, sound, or form.

seem possibly correct. That is why research is an adventure.

The object of the whole enterprise is to *describe* nature.[5] At first it seems wise, at all events it seems to have been universally customary, to describe natural phenomena so as to group them. That makes description easier because there result fewer descriptions. Classification is what this phase of the undertaking is called. Sometimes, especially in our day, there lurks, unfortunately, something invidious in the remark that an investigator is merely "describing." Descriptions must naturally be exact. Exactness can in fact be exhibited, purely and deliberately, without quantitative expression in descriptions of things as they occur in nature, rough and in the whole. Men who have carried on this phase of natural inquiry have been known as naturalists or, at a stage more organized, more complicated, systematists. Hippocrates, Pliny, Linnæus, Sydenham, Darwin, Lyell, Audubon, Wheeler, form such a group. Their very names are proof that nothing derogatory attaches to their interests or their methods. Without labors like theirs, there can be no natural science. Without them we should be talking of phenixes, unicorns, and other mythological animals. It is an evidence of the literalness of the culture of the Greeks that, unlike Egyptians or

[5] There are those to whom action appears a more impressive and compelling motive than description. The object of the enterprise would then be to accomplish an end. The difference may be essential but it may also be a difference in emphasis. If astronomy began in the interests of action, it has remained a means to satisfy mere curiosity; or, is it perhaps to return to its original function?

Orientals, they entered little into nature faking. The objects of concern to scientists have been natural objects. Later—and later may be taken to have a chronological meaning, though it may have also a logical one—when the *experimental era* began in its modern form, reliance came to be placed, not by any means exclusively but accompanied by a certain glamour which obscured the relations among methods, on the experimental method. A powerful agent for extending knowledge became available. The experimental method involves the conception that comprehension of a thing, of a phenomenon, can be furthered powerfully by dissecting it, by pulling it apart, by measuring and by weighing and by counting.[6] I need not dwell on what is universally known, the extraordinary and unbelievable success of the method. By it Galilei, Harvey, Newton, Young, Lavoisier, their modern equally great successors, and an enormous host of followers, have enriched modern thought, modern knowledge, and modern life.

When the experimental era began in its modern form, the temptation was great to believe that once the parts were known, the whole would be comprehended. It was another way of thinking that the whole is equal to the sum of the parts. But doubt began to assail thinkers that matters were not so simple. It was the same situation that confronted the King's

[6] It needs scarcely to be pointed out that what is called synthesis, as in the preparation of chemical substances, dyes, for example, or aromatic compounds, or in metallurgy when new alloys are made, or in technical procedures, or advances in general, is an extension merely of the analytical process.

horses and the King's men when they tried, after his great fall, to put Humpty Dumpty together again. The attempt did not work. Because it did not and because in a very widespread manner there is current conviction that it cannot, the idea has been put forward by S. Alexander, Lloyd Morgan, A. N. Whitehead, and General Smuts that, in putting things together again after they have been taken apart, something new becomes ingredient, something not in the constituent elements. It is, to use a crude example, as if $2 + 2$ did not quite equal 4, that to attain 4, something not in the synthesist's hands or mind, entered into the new composition. The doctrine that something new occurs has come to be known as emergent evolution. In speaking of analysis and research, it is unnecessary to lay undue emphasis on the imperfections of the analytical process, but it is desirable to be alive to their existence so as to avoid the disappointments which otherwise are almost inescapable. There have, in point of fact, been a goodly number. Leaving aside the emergence of new qualities, a phase after all of synthesis, the delays which have taken place in the cures of infectious diseases, like tuberculosis, like typhoid fever, like poliomyelitis, after the discovery and identification of the agents that help to occasion them, are known to everybody.

The whole adventure, classification and analysis, is science. To repeat, it has two aspects, the natural phenomena themselves and a way of looking. Of the way of looking, there has just been discussion. Of the natural phenomena, there is something to say concerning a significant difference between medical and other natural sciences, the difference to which I wished to direct attention and which I wish briefly to weigh. It is the *enduring interest* that attaches to other natural sciences in contrast with the medical ones. Consider such interests as the origin of species, the origin of astronomical systems, matter, heat, electricity, the formation of the earth, light, heredity. These are concerns as little influenced as may be by time and place. There was never a time when they did not engage serious intellectual attention; they do so now; there is good reason to believe they will continue to do so. These phenomena awoke, and continue to awake, enduring interests because they are enduring objects.

Turn next to the situation in the study of diseases. I have been dwelling on enduringness in interest in the objects of natural science because the objects studied in these sciences are themselves enduring. Now diseases, whether of plants or of animals, no matter what their nature, are statistically something extra.[7] They are occurrences which, in subtle or coarse ways, change the usual behavior of living things. The organisms are said to suffer, hence the use of the word, in the British sense, pathology. Beside being

[7] Extra, not anticipated in a state of "health." I do not mean that process "a" is joined to organism "b" and that a + b constitute a disease. In this sense "a" would be what has been called an entity, an "ens." That is far from my meaning. "Extra" describes the whole organism, exhibiting phenomena, not counted as occurring in health. Health itself is a statistical conception.

something extra, their becoming established in a society is not permanent. They change with time, they change with locality. The sweating sickness is gone. How long poliomyelitis may have existed is not known. Diseases devastating in the tropics do not exist in the temperate zones. In other cases, like rheumatic fever, the reverse may be true. Diseases may continue to turn out to be transient sojourners. By paying a necessary price, there are diseases of which we can rid ourselves, for example, syphilis, perhaps scarlet fever, no doubt a number of others. Diseases, furthermore, have no independent existence; they are recognized when they have transformed the nature of their hosts, plant or animal, temporarily or permanently.

If, as I have been surmising, enduringness is a characteristic of things which have become constituted objects of study in natural sciences, it seems apparent that diseases do not partake of that quality. That is clearly the case in infectious diseases. Nor in all probability do chemical diseases, of which the deficiency states are examples, such as pellagra, pernicious anemia, rickets, and scurvy. Another group of diseases of great importance may be designated physiological. Physiology may be termed the study of the living behavior of an organism, as different from its mere structure. In the study of diseases, the physiology of an animal has importance because it occupies a place like the study of metallurgy in the mechanism of a steam engine. But a disease is not merely quantitatively changed physiology. A disease is something

over and above and therefore different from this. The
place of physiology in this scheme must not be confused. Physiology undertakes the analysis of something, animal or plant, reasonably long enduring in a
species or a genus—the circulation, reproduction, digestion. These are mechanisms which are neither
temporary nor local. There are, of course, physiological derangements which are usually called diseases,
eclampsia being an example, or perhaps a certain
variety of arterial hypertension, or fibrillation of the
auricles of the heart, or psychogenic hyperthyroidism.
And a special case is that of senescence, the aging
through which we all pass. My case as to enduringness is naturally not as clear-cut in respect to physiological occurrences as the distinction I have drawn
suggests. Evolution and the disappearance of species
and genera see to that. But there is enough of background for this distinction to occasion the social consequence in which can be perceived implications of
great importance to the position the study of medicine occupies.[8]

8 There is a point of view from which contributions to general
knowledge result from the study of ephemeral phenomena or from
acquaintance with transient experience. Contributions so derived
can, no doubt, exert significant influence in developing insights,
conceptions, and procedures which come much later to fruition.
Broad intellectual streams can originate in obscure rills. But there
remains, nevertheless, a value which enduringness, as a method of
characterization, can be made to possess. Even so, as a characteristic,
it is unnecessary to assume that it has more than relative value.
Were diseases dependent on a relation to bacteria wholly to disappear, bacteriology, for example, having received its great stimulus
from this association, may be expected to remain an important interest nevertheless, because of the growing place it is coming to occupy in agriculture and elsewhere.

The use of another word can now be examined. The word *empiricism* provides an opportunity for examining certain ideas and procedures commonly employed in natural science. When a certain amount of animadversion is intended in the use of the word, the adjective "crude" is prefixed. This phrase, "crude empiricism," has been used especially with reference to the study of diseases, the assumption being that the study of diseases is something apart, in fact, from other studies of natural phenomena, something perhaps a little backward. On more careful reflection it becomes clear that "crude empiricism" is a phrase universally applicable to a level of discovery at which what is called "thinking" has not been much employed or, cannot be, either in the existing state of knowledge or by the individuals who indulge in that occupation. Now, when what is called "crude empiricism" is exhibited, the subject matter under investigation is relatively in a raw, native state and the means which are used to analyze that subject matter are not, in comparison with what is possible elsewhere, or in some other discipline, of a sort to be called refined. An example in medicine is the use of quinine in malaria before an insight into the nature of malaria or the composition of quinine was obtained. Syphilis and mercury is another example, or dropsy and digitalis. In physical science, telephony and the nature of electricity, though a very rough analogue, may serve as example. The form in which I have stated this situation suggests its meaning. When something is done or some interference with a system is undertaken, as in the examples just given, it is in the natural organized state of the material, the crude, native state, in which the operation is performed. There exists no guide, furthermore, to suggest what form the operation should take. If malaria is not known to be protozoal in origin, or if it is unknown that the infecting agent is susceptible to quinine, but a therapeutic attempt is made, none the less, that attempt is empirical and may be termed crude. That it should be so is in the nature of things. If the object is to understand anything whatever, a beginning must be, or is, made. Once a beginning is made, successive efforts at understanding, if on the road to success, become less and less "crude." In the case of matter, electricity, energy, methods of analysis have now become so refined that it is evident how long a distance has been traveled from rubbing cat's fur on amber (electron). The more we analyze, the further investigation becomes removed from crudity. Because analysis has taken place in successive simple stages; because, covering the heart of a phenomenon, there are layers of impenetrability like the layers of petals covering the heart of an artichoke, as Sherrington was moved to say; because that is the way an experimenter must look at the world; behind each mechanism is hidden another mechanism. Obviously the metaphor of the artichoke is imperfect—there is a last layer of leaves, small and apparently confused in arrangement, and then the heart. But in the phenomena to which scientists devote themselves, who knows when the last petal has been plucked and the heart of a natural process uncovered? There is a chance here (and the man who knows how to take it is the artist in science) that for *an* object, it is unnecessary—no, destructive in fact—to go further than a certain point, the point being the emergent level for which search was being made. Protection against pneumonia will not, by way of illustration, be solved at the atomic level. If the appropriate level is passed, the nature of the thing sought may elude one's grasp. Hawthorne's story of the birthmark and beauty tells the story of the devastation wrought by a perfectionist.

Whether knowledge is empirical depends often on the standpoint of the critic. A molecule, a protein molecule, may seem very refined in comparison with a man, but to an electron it looks enormously complex. The whole business is relative.

The point about empiricism and crudeness requires no further laboring. It must be apparent that at the beginning nothing else than crudeness is possible. Later on more insight may have been gained, but the term still be applicable. Were the case of causation simple, as it is not, it would be possible to prescribe how a situation must be analyzed and possible to prophesy the results. There is little confidence nowadays that that can be the situation anywhere. Further understanding depends therefore on trial and error in the choice of analytical technics. Since that is inescapable all scientific analysis is crude and all knowledge empirical. The only point of view from which empirical knowledge is less crude depends on the amount of relevant research that has been made. Much more has become known about malaria and syphilis, about quinine and mercury, about dropsy and digitalis, about energy and electrons. But to him who confronts a choice of the next step, the situation contains elements of crudity which he recognizes as not far removed from that of that predecessor of his who took the adventurous first step. So long as there are further steps there is adventure and so long as there is adventure, there is crudity. Otherwise research would be a commonplace procession along the avenues of the known. The Lindberghs would be the last to underestimate the Nungessers.

He who tells us we must halt a research until analysis has proceeded further must be certain of a number of matters around which this discussion has taken place. He must know that further analysis of a complex situation is rewarding. A chemist preparing therapeutic agents will appreciate this point. Suppose it were optochin he had prepared and were told that too frequently giving his preparation caused blindness. Against pneumococci his agent worked admirably, that was his original objective. To perfect his agent and to safeguard it against unexpected, unfortunate consequence, what must he do? Must he search for other substances, similar in structure, must he try another group of agents, or must he, by analyzing optochin further, hope to discover what is offending in the structure of his drug at a different lower level of organization?

Quinine and quinidine afford another example.

The auricles, the entrance chambers in the hearts of human beings, often lose their custom of orderly contraction and, do what we call, fibrillate, a state in which they live and act but do so in a very disorderly fashion. A sufferer from this disorder once noticed that frequently when he took quinine, the normal behavior of his heart was restored. He narrated his experience to his physician in Vienna, Professor Wenckebach. Professor Wenckebach sought to repeat his patient's attempts but met with scant success, and told this story in one of his treatises. It occurred to another physician, Frey, to try more or less systematically other chemical substances with which quinine is related. At this point it becomes necessary, perhaps unwarrantedly, to assume certain biographical details. Was that a rational procedure of Frey's, was there good reason to think other quinine-like substances would work better than quinine; if so, which one, related how to quinine? Or should he explore other substances, not quinine but substances belonging to that series? Or should he attempt to build up quinine into a drug more complex? Or should he break it down to find what in quinine actually worked in Professor Wenckebach's patient, in short, purify the drug? Or should he look for a substance which, in Professor Wenckebach's patient, aided quinine but was absent in his own? Or did his own patient harbor a substance which interfered with the action of quinine? All these were possibilities. A complete account of how Frey behaved in this situation is unknown, it usually is. He may have tried none of these or many. He had a single guide only. He was told quinine worked in a *single* person. We are speaking of levels of organization. The only point of immediate concern is whether he should have analyzed further to find a simpler substance. It may be, he should have done so, for the result of his labors has been effective in about sixty per cent only of patients. In that sense the problem is still open and the various choices enumerated for investigation still available. What Frey did was to explore what is possible on the very level of organization of quinine sulphate. He found in the group a substance which worked sixty per cent of the time, quinidine sulphate, identical with quinine sulphate except for its action on polarized light. This was turned left, quinine turns it right. The structural formula symbolizes the difference in that the two are written as mirror images of each other. In this case, no further analytical procedures were undertaken. Success, partial, it is true, came on a level of organization no different from before. There was no way of knowing beforehand that this would be the case. Attention to causation would not have helped. It was not known, it is not known now, what causally is essential in this reaction. It is therefore unprofitable to search for it.

It is in the nature of things that students of any phenomenon must have first-hand knowledge of that phenomenon itself. For simple description first-hand acquaintance is all that is requisite. For analysis it is essential in addition, to possess knowledge of the art and practise of appropriate forms of analysis. There is no fundamental difference in the nature of these procedures for students of diseases and for other natural scientists. Nor is there a difference in the operations which the mind undertakes. The intellectual powers appropriate to elucidation of the two are the same, whether the object of study is a disease or an electron. The physical methods employed in laboratories naturally differ and are especially adapted to the objectives and material being analyzed. But the mind proceeds always in the same way; it knows few tricks and these few it employs indifferently wherever it has use for them. When it comes to procedure, the mental act, indifferent to rational objective, measures length or volume or frequency. The behavior of the mind remains always the same irrespective of the tools it causes to be used in the various situations in which it acts—it describes, it classifies, it dissects. Experience must come first and then the analysis of that experience, whatever the object.

But a potential difference exists nevertheless. The practise of medicine is an ancient calling. It is as intricate as it is ancient. It is one of the nicest of the arts. Its practitioners have been in the habit of performing many social functions. These have been so absorbing that until almost contemporary time neither leisure nor opportunity nor perhaps desire was available to proceed beyond simple description, of which there has been much, to analysis [9] which has but recently, and let us hope not tentatively, begun.

[9] Not psycho-analysis.

What needs appreciating is that the gap between practise and analyzing is by way of being bridged. The existence of the gap cannot be ignored. Of its deterring effect much has been made—in my judgment much too much. When students were inadequately, or not at all, trained for research, more weight attached to the exclusive demands of practise than now. Much has changed, not least, the estimate placed on traditional knowledge and on practical legerdemain though medical opinion still insists upon transmitting a great deal of this in formal education. But in spite of all change, of persons interested in diseases, two types can be seen to emerge, one interested in advancing knowledge about them, and the other in treating them. The difference is similar to that between engineers and physicists. Physicians who wish to learn how to analyze, now can do so, and do so to extraordinarily useful purpose. But there is the difficulty I have mentioned, the gap. It is real and it is important. It occasions a difference not found, I fancy, to the same extent in other sciences having both theoretical and practical phases. Who would suppose, for example, that Graves disease (exophthalmic goiter), in order properly to be comprehended, requires knowledge of physiological occurrences and chemical processes obviously not necessarily within the competent knowledge of conscientious practitioners of medicine? Or in the kind of cardiac affection common in older individuals, insight into and control of the most intimate behavior of muscle fibers? And not only that, but knowledge of what underlies the behavior of those muscle fibers and their ability to carry on work. I have mentioned other difficulties which beset physicians, but here is a major one. To treat what is so obviously wrong, he must have learned, in physiology and physics and chemistry, what a man can learn only, if he learn it at all, as the result of the expenditure of all his energy. Research, in these circumstances, was at an impasse. For twenty-five years and more the effort has been made to bridge this gap by providing opportunity for a few physicians at least, to free themselves from the demands of practice. The divorce of research from demands so continuously absorbing has accomplished noteworthy results. Whether the divorce is adequate has not, I think, received sufficient scrutiny.

This much can be said safely, that time for research has been gained. And this in addition, that to concentrate effort a certain amount of irrelevant information may be left at the wayside. And finally this, that physicians who observe the phenomena of diseases receive from their intimate contact with patients and their ailments, stimuli to ferret out the meaning of what they observe. No one else has access to that knowledge. Having that knowledge and requisite training, the hope is still entertained that physicians, specially chosen, can solve the relevant problems. It would be idle to underrate the difficulties. They do not so much consist in translating problems from bedside to laboratory as from transvaluing one pattern of knowledge with its technical (clinical) apparatus to another quite different pattern with equally exacting, if not more complicated, technical (mechanical) apparatus. To recognize, for example, a cardiac disease, to think of its origin, to study its future, is obviously a different enterprise from search for the mechanism of the contraction of muscle on which its clinical manifestations depend. For that search involves far away knowledge of proteins and the part they play in the complex structure of muscle, as a result of which they contract. Other illustrations may be chosen—syphilis for example, its dependence on a micro-organism, a spirochæte, and the susceptibility of spirochætes to poisoning by arsenical compounds. Or still another, diabetes mellitus, depending essentially on destruction or malfunction of a single structure in the pancreas, the islands of Langerhans, and its remediability on a substance extracted from these islands.

This discussion and these illustrations should suffice to define a peculiar situation in medical science. I have already mentioned a special characteristic of the subject matter of "medicine," the absence of "enduringness" exhibited by diseases. And now I have added illustrations dealing with the apparently wide interval between diseases as natural phenomena and the cumbersome traditional technic for learning about them—the practical aspects of this study, on the one hand, and the equipment necessary to deal with the analytical procedures necessary in research, on the other—to explain how the position of medical science and of medical scientists has come to be somewhat different from that in other sciences and how the intellectual position of medical scientists has been regarded as differing from that of other scientists.

It is, I think, impossible just now to exaggerate from a public point of view the importance of treatment. The motives which have brought great funds for study into existence have not, except in connection with great dangers, arisen from general public interest. The year 1776 was remarkable, aside from having witnessed the signature of the Declaration of Independence, for the effort Johann Peter Frank made on behalf of the Archbishop of Speyer to gather information on a social, political, or, at all events, on a grand, scale, concerning the health of a population so as to make this more secure. That adventure began an epoch. Usually it has been the illness of a friend or a member of a family that stimulated the insistent interest of private philanthropists. The universities had no funds. Government took a minimum interest only.

Once, when I defined medicine as the study of *diseases,* Doctor Thayer objected vigorously because in his judgment, joined inseparably to the study of diseases, was the need to get on with the business of curing these diseases. The term medicine, he thought, included both. Obviously a term can mean whatever we say that it does. There is no reason against the use of the term "medicine" in the manner on which Doctor Thayer insisted. It is preferable though, I think, not to make the meaning of terms too inclusive; that is a way of obscuring the variety of aspects which a situation can be made to disclose. It is undoubted, indeed in the world of medicine the notion is widespread, that to search out the nature of diseases is one of our chief obligations. But there is no doubt also, that the notion of curing diseases is universally believed to be a function of physicians. The function of medicine in the *cure* of diseases is so deeply imbedded in both public and professional minds that there have been periods of impatience with the belief that the business of curing is difficult and complicated (Hahnemann, and others) and with those who insisted on an education more or less elaborate for men whose office it might become to search out cures. Joining the search for knowledge of diseases with curing has, I think, tended to obscure the problems presented by both. It is not without importance to point out that to make cures provides, within properly defined limits, for a kind of activity not encountered in other disciplines.

Cures are of two kinds—we have depended on what I have been calling "crude empiricism" for one of them. Here there is no use for the refinement of analytical procedures. Agents not rationally related to complaints are used to mitigate them. Such agents do turn up, as digitalis in the case of dropsy, suggested by a Shropshire housewife who interested the willing Dr. Withering in her experiences; or when, owing to faith in the providence of God, the notion is entertained that where diseases occur, there in close proximity are their cures to be found, as salicylic acid (the willow) in the case of rheumatic fever.

The other kind of cure relies on nothing so simple, nothing so fortuitous. In this case cures are conceived possible because of a belief that there exists something in a morbid condition, central to it, a knowledge of which would further the possibility of cure, as of micro-organisms in typhoid fever; or of toxins in diphtheria; or excess activity of an organ, as in thyroid hyperactivity; or deficiency in a secretion, as in pernicious anemia; or defect or destruction in tissues or organs exerting either immediate or remote consequences, as the effect on the heart in beri-beri or of the late result of rheumatic fever; or, following in the footsteps of Ponce de Leon, substances which neutralize the action of agents that make the body age.

But how are such substances to be found? There must be no mistake; they are actually and feverishly being sought. The sciences of chemotherapy, physicotherapy, immunology, pharmacology, the founding of institutes for the study of cancer and for this, that, or the other, are evidence of the liveliness of the quest. Sometimes the direction of research is simple enough, the agents being already well known; in the case of hemolytic streptococcus infections, sulphanilamide; in tetanus, tetanus antitoxin; in the failure of cardiac muscle, digitalis. But in the case of cancer the situation is different; since neither cause nor cure is known, shall the search be for an agent to combat a virus or some other substance or for the correction of a constitutional arrangement responsible for the licentious growth? The direction which the search is to take is often the subject of sharp cleavages of opinion. The single subject, cancer, illustrates how in the process of analysis, talents, equipments, trainings of different forms may become serviceable. If you believe cancer is caused by a virus you want men to search for it who are perhaps differently endowed and certainly differently equipped from men who believe the solution of this problem lies in discovering, as responsible for its origin or development, a chemical substance to be neutralized.

To a choice of means, beside haphazard, there is no other guide but reason. But reason operates in the domain of causation and its tool is logic informed by insight which in an exact sense, is experience in action. Now, as has long been evident, reason alone is inadequate. Hope resides in the use of reason to limit the region of investigation so that then, within narrow, indeed within the narrowest framework possible, systematic trial and error can be attempted. If science is empiric, somehow experience provides it with a pattern. That is Aristotelian. Here is the inescapable region for the display of scholarship, ingenuity, resource. What the issue is to be in seeking the cause or cure of cancer, no one now, I presume, would be bold enough to declare. It is a fortunate circumstance that men of many minds, everywhere, are engaged in this search. But the point to be made is that once the method of crude empiricism is abandoned, the alternative, which is analysis, requires technical education not at the disposal of every one interested in a subject. The problem is the problem of the physician as scientist. Special training is the price of analysis and analysis is the consequence of the failure of the obvious.

I could have drawn this lesson on rational therapeutics from another source. It has been said, and said plentifully, that the dawning interest in ailments of the aging is the result of social pressure. Formerly that pressure was exercised, as now in the case of poliomyelitis, to secure protection from bacterial diseases because they, often being contagious, were dangerous and required quarantine. Comparable pressure is being exercised now because the ailments incident to older age are long drawn out and tend to be costly, indeed, very costly. The study of statistics created awareness of this situation; deaths from certain causes were increasing. In the course of a few years a general conception of what this meant began to be clear, or clearer. Little was known. The study of aging began then in a more serious fashion.

The problem what and how to study is not, in some respects, unlike that in cancer. What causes aging? Is it necessary or preventable? If preventable, does it result from subtle injuries inflicted in the course of ordinary living, injuries due to infection or diet or to other environmental moments? Where is evidence to be sought? In changes in the arteries or in some other tissue or organ? Is its cause a substance secreted within the organism, constituting a master reaction, not by design, though that is not an unusual conception, but because of its fortuitous and unavoidable nature? If aging is the result of any of these causes, obviously means to bring the process to a standstill can conceivably be found. But if it should turn out that it is none of these or none comparable to them, that aging is universal, it will be necessary to turn to the notion that aging takes place in the nature of things, that somehow it is incident to living, an expression of the togetherness of the organism, not a follow-the-leader mechanism; that the disabilities and ailments to which it gives rise call for alleviation of disability and suffering, different, or perhaps not different, from those that are sought on the assumption of preventability.

From the point of view of research, the meaning is clear. The resources of intelligence are wanted badly in this situation, natural historians, statisticians, morphologists, chemists of several sorts, physiologists, physicians. There may be short cuts to discoveries in this category, but the history of science does not encourage us to expect to find one. It is more likely that in order to learn what to do, it is necessary first to search out the forces that are at work and the precise forms they assume. Attempts to anticipate solutions by short cuts have too often been futile. We are, naturally, not told that enough is known to make a solution possible. And then it is no longer believed widely that genius can advance far beyond current knowledge. Newton, for example, is unthinkable as a contemporary of Aristotle. Failure in scientific research is often the natural answer to premature adventure. The frequency of simultaneous discoveries is evidence for the correctness of this view. Pressing on the door of the unknown is nowadays constantly taking place. But we do not believe we know beforehand who will force an entrance. We believe, therefore, in freedom of research, one of the academic freedoms which ought accordingly, sedulously to be preserved. Whether a research can be made to pay, is a matter of judgment. Who has this judgment? Experience counts, of course, though the inexperienced, like Parsifal, often see the light. But Aristotle, Harvey, Young, Helmholtz, Pasteur, Hering, Ludwig, Gaskell, Darwin, to name only biologists, were not inexperienced. Since chance enters the calculation, there is little room for dogma.

The clinic has been an integral part in the scheme for providing for the care and study of patients and their ailments. The very fact that clinics present the opportunity of seeing and comparing the manifestations exhibited by patients has facilitated greatly, as Shryock has pointed out, the description and classification of diseases. To be able to do this is, as we now know, indispensable in the development of scientific knowledge. When the stage of analyzing the appearances of diseases is reached, the equipment possible to clinics is essential. Equipment includes, for example, laboratories for chemical analyses, for the study of the physiological and physical aspects of diseases, for bacteriology, serology, immunity, hematology. In the past hundred years, but more especially in the past thirty, such opportunities have actually been provided on a fair scale. It has become possible for physicians to study whatever phase of a disease seems important. Naturally clinics do not neglect the management of patients. On the contrary. They exist for the sole purpose of encouraging better and proper treatment, as adequate as contemporary knowledge permits. It is illuminating to observe how quickly the general public has learned to find its way to university clinics in the belief that the latest information on the cure of diseases is to be found there, where the search for their causes and nature is actively going on. The fear, once entertained, that patients dread examinations by students and are unwilling to subject themselves to novel procedures even though undertaken with proper precautions, has been found not to exist or to have been much exaggerated. How to carry on clinical research is one of the lessons which has been learned.

Now, what can be successfully undertaken in the way of research in clinics depends on several factors. It is obvious that the subjects for research are diseases which the patients in a clinic present, these being presumably representative of the forms of illness present in a community. Certain illnesses can be profitably studied, others not. It would for example have been futile for Borelli or for von Helmont in the seventeenth and eighteenth centuries to study infectious diseases. Underlying and contributory knowledge was not yet available.

In the choice of subjects, what I have been calling the level of organization counts, and counts heavily. A distinguished biologist of the past generation spoke often to his friends of the uselessness of investigating diseases until more was known about the behavior of cells, the ultimate proximate constituents composing animals and plants. In certain directions his view was undoubtedly sound. But sera, like those used successfully in treating certain pneumonias or in diphtheria, or a drug like quinidine, or bacteria as causes of diseases, or fibrillation of the auricles as underlying a striking disorder of the heart beat, all these can be, have been, and are being, studied to the great benefit of man without carrying on the investigation at a level of organization much below that on which the going concern which is the organism, carries on. It goes without saying that every analysis occurs on a level simpler than that of the thing analyzed. That is in the inescapable nature of analysis. But how far below? I have been saying, not very far, because relevant knowledge is usually not available; and in the solution of a problem, a level too far below may cease to be relevant. In analyzing morbid processes, the opportunity should be available to carry on an investigation at that level precisely where an experienced or an especially gifted person decides it may be profitable.

Objection is raised on occasion to affording this opportunity in clinics, the point being that that opportunity should be sought elsewhere either because elsewhere the cost, financially, may be less; or because the inclusion elsewhere of that research may be more appropriate; or because historically there is value in retaining that study at the locus of its origin. But this is a workaday world; it is difficult to get things done anywhere; men carry on, each his own business and do that with difficulty and against odds. Answers are sought because they are needed. Pathological anatomists, for example, are often in despair because of the lacunæ, of great importance to them, left by anatomists. The situation is exactly similar when clinicians require information not supplied by physiologists. But even if anatomists and physiologists have developed a subject, there can be no obligation upon them to go on with it. They may not be aware of the need of a next step. To those to whom taking it is necessary, it is scant comfort to know where preliminary investigations were carried on, if they are no longer being housed there. The fructification of ideas cannot be shackled to a building or even to a locality. But even if the study of a subject is duplicated, the loss is usually not great. Identity in result is rare, mutual criticism is profitable, slight differences in procedure are desirable.

There must, of course, be some sort of common sense on what is investigated in clinics; no one now would regard it as sensible to establish a laboratory for the study of electrons. But such researches as on the metabolism of bacteria, on nomograms describing acid-base and other equilibria, the location and behavior of salts and water, the mechanism of respiratory ferments, and no doubt a host of others, seem to be appropriate. To afford hospitality in clinics for such studies seems wholly reasonable. So will domiciling other activities when the principles involved are scrutinized and understood, such as describing long-drawn-out diseases and senescent states, especially when the interest in them is peculiar to the clinic and the emphasis necessarily different from that outside.

The question finally arises as to whether men exist in clinics willing to devote themselves to investigations at fundamental levels. Though enterprises at such levels are relatively new, it appears already that little or no difficulty is being experienced. If there is difficulty it exists perhaps in the temptation to draw to too practical purposes the labors of those who should be studying at simpler levels. But if so-called fundamental researches are fostered, there exists the possibility of guiding them within pragmatic limits and of acquainting clinicians with the value of such enterprses. Against the cost, if the cost is high, must be balanced the motives, the interest in, the concern for the subject. It seems too theoretical to expel from clinics what can be done there profitably, especially when a clinical interest meets with no outside echo. There are things, it seems, more expensive than money.

The discussion on the nature of the medical clinic has not, I believe, these many years past, given due place to these more general aspects of its life. Primary attention was focused on practise and on teaching because they seemed to be more urgent. These three, teaching, practise, and research can, of course, be conducted as coördinate functions. The devotion to practise and to teaching must in no sense be whittled away. But it will not be if the experience of recent years is a guide. What is wanted is a realization that in university clinics, all scholars need not be cut according to the same pattern. Traditionally the rôles of teacher and practitioner have been emphasized, perhaps overemphasized. But a clinic affords opportunity for the display of diverse talents; there can be doubt no longer that men of diverse talents can find happiness and opportunity there. To arrive at the precise specifications should not, within this framework, be too difficult. If the conviction begins to prevail that these various functions should find their home there, their adjustment and accommodation may safely be left to the slow, one would hope not too slow, processes of time.

The crucial point appears to be that, to succeed, research in medicine must be regarded a serious undertaking. For whatever reasons, the issues are now regarded as sufficiently urgent by the general public, so that government is devoting increasing attention to the health of the community. To take this problem seriously means that scholars in medicine must be permitted to be serious, as are those in other callings. Education and the equipment for research must, of course, be adequate. And the rewards for service must be ample. Free and frequent criticism must be cultivated. This has been sharp in a technological sense. Experimental nonsense is not lightly tolerated. From a more general point of view, that dealing with the purposes and direction of research, criticism seems to be less well informed. Criticism of a kind can be found in presidential addresses but the vigor, insight, and fearlessness displayed is perhaps not sufficiently incisive.

This is what I understand the meaning of medical research to be. The study of diseases has been separated in a category somewhat different from that of the other sciences. That has been due in part to the nature of its subject matter, being in a limited sense, less enduring than that taken for analysis in the other sciences. It has been due in part also to the lateness with which analytical methods have been employed in the study of diseases. The use of them now is in full swing but, being new, the education of men eager to employ them has not been adequately conceived to this end. For this reason also, a critical approach to the analysis of diseases has not yet fully evolved.

Of the objects of human interest, diseases are far from the least. The need for getting on with the understanding of many maladies is urgent. These are very varied, and require for their elucidation professional insight and equipment of a high order. The problems are becoming not less, but more intricate, the more the methods of empiricism change from crude to less crude. The meaning of medical research is to understand the mechanisms at play and to be concerned with their alleviation and cure.

III

DR. WATSON AND
MR. SHERLOCK HOLMES

BY

HARRISON STANFORD MARTLAND, M.D.
PROFESSOR OF FORENSIC MEDICINE, NEW YORK UNIVERSITY
COLLEGE OF MEDICINE

III

DR. WATSON AND MR. SHERLOCK HOLMES

I

I ON THE EVOLUTION AND FUTURE OF DETECTIVE AND
MYSTERY FICTION FROM ÆSOP TO EDGAR ALLAN POE

"DETECTIVE stories," as we know them, must arise from the social consciousness of the importance of the individual death which results in investigation, study, and solution. However, among the ancients, history reveals but little interest in individual fatalities. Police powers were entirely relegated to the soldiery, whose chief interest, in common with the populace, was the exploration and exploitation of new lands. Although no "detective stories," as such, have come down to us, many instances in ancient literature reveal deductions of great detective ability. Perhaps one of the earliest exists in Æsop's *Fables* (620-560 B.C.). In the fable of the lion and the fox we find the following: "Why do you not come to pay your respects to me?" Æsop's lion asked the fox. "I beg your majesty's pardon," replied the fox, "But I noticed the track of the animals that have already come to you; and, while I see many hoof-marks going in, I see none coming out. Till the animals that have entered your cave come out again, I prefer to remain in the open air." This is apparently the first mention of the importance of foot-prints in the detection of crime.

Even during the Middle Ages there was no adequate police organization and the tales of the populace centered about heroes and war gods rather than the solution of crime. Murder, poisoning, rape, all flourished but retribution was personal and in the form of the feud.

In the literature of the sixteenth and seventeenth centuries there are almost no stories which focus the attention on the activities of the representatives of law and order. To the contrary, most tales glorify the brigand and ridicule such officers of law enforcement as existed at that time. This is particularly true in the literature of the Mediterranean countries.

During the eighteenth century most of the national boundaries of the Old World were more or less fixed, and the people were thus enabled to turn attention from warfare to their local social problems. With the organization of the metropolitan police systems, we note the development of real detective fiction, the first evidence of which we find in England in the pre-Victorian period. These facts plus the natural inborn respect of the English for law and order make that country the logical birth-place of detective fiction as we know it. Subsequently, although the greater portion of that type of writing has come from Anglo-Saxon authors, many examples of good detective fiction and mystery stories are to be found in the French and German literature.

EDGAR ALLAN POE

It is to an American, however, that we must accredit the development of both the plot and the typical detective found in our contemporary detective and mystery fiction.

Poe, the son of an actress, was born in Boston in 1809. Two years later both of Poe's parents died and left three destitute children. Edgar was adopted by one John Allan, a prosperous tobacco merchant of Richmond, Virginia, at the request of his childless wife. During childhood, Poe was spoiled, and was apparently led to believe that he would inherit Allan's fortune. Poe was well educated and attended schools both in England and Virginia. He was a good athlete. While a student at the University of Virginia, Poe developed a passion for gambling and drinking, which was to handicap him for life. He left the University, enlisted and served two years in the army (when under orders Poe could be a diligent and capable subordinate). He then entered West Point, where he remained aloof and was not well liked by his fellow cadets. He lasted about one year, when he was courtmartialed and expelled. Allan at this time disinherited Poe and left him nothing. Most of the rest of Poe's life was spent in Baltimore with his paternal aunt, Mrs. Clemm, who was his protector and supporter, in so far as her poverty would permit.

During the early years of this period he developed as a poet, writer of fiction and critic.

Poe, throughout most of his later life, was undoubtedly a chronic alcoholic. He has been greatly maligned, however, for he was not drunk all the time, but rather suffered attacks of periodic acute alcoholism—dipsomania. Poe was highly neurotic, had a psychopathic personality, and probably disturbances of the psyche. Surges of suppressed and unhappy emotions into the consciousness were apparently often of such intensity and character as to be well nigh intolerable. At times, especially when sober, as he often was for considerable periods, Poe was gentle, revealed good breeding, and was an indefatigable worker. In 1849 Poe died, when but forty years of age.

The Three Dupin Stories. In the so-called *Dupin stories,*[1] Poe introduces an eccentric, brilliant, private detective, Chevalier C. Auguste Dupin. The introduction of a private detective who outclasses the police and other officials in his observations and deductions pleases the reader, for the public has always cherished a mild contempt for the police—the "flat-footed, dumb copper."

This technic has been imitated by authors ever since—Philo Vance, Nero Wolfe, and so on—and has been literally worn out. With the more modern scientific methods in the detection of crime, police inves-

[1] For the evolution of the plot and the detective I am greatly indebted to Dorothy L. Sayers' classical treatment of the subject. Those interested should read her introduction in the book *The Omnibus of Crime* (New York, Payson and Clarke, Ltd., 1929).

tigators are coming into their own and the character
of the private detective is on the way out.

Poe introduces a narrator to tell his stories. An admiring and "thick-headed" friend. In this technic the
narrator becomes a "stooge." [2] The reader thus de-
lights in thinking he is a little more ingenious and
intelligent than the narrator—"I spotted that," and
so on. The stooge can eulogize the detective to the
blue canopy of the heavens without embarrassment.
By describing clues as presented to the stooge, the
author preserves an attitude of frankness—of laying
all the cards on the table—at the same time withholding the special knowledge upon which depends the
proper interpretation of the clues. As a result mystery
and interest are kept up until the end.

In "The Mystery of Marie Roget," Dupin solves
the disappearance and murder of a shop-girl. This is
done by analysis and deductions from newspaper clip-
pings, based upon a true story of the disappearance
of one Mary Cecilia Rogers in New York. This story
is classified by Sayers as of the classic or intellectual

[2] The development of the "stooge" started a few years ago with
the catch-as-catch-can comedian, the late Ted Healy. It is said
(New York *Times*) that one afternoon in 1921, while appearing in
vaudeville in Brooklyn, Healy suddenly found that four or five of
his stage associates had fled. No whit dismayed, he snatched his
valet and two friends from his dressing room. The performance was
completed ad lib, with Healy doing all the talking and making capital of his comrades' embarrassment. Thereafter the gang of Healy's
"stooges," known originally as his "racketeers," were the indestruct-
ible martyrs on whose shoulders he mounted to fame. In the *Dictionary of American Slang*, "stooge" denotes a stage fool or butt of
all jokes. The "stooge act" is at present very popular on the radio,
in the movies and on the stage.

type—such stories illustrate analytical ingenuity and allow the reader to try his own deductions, but are often dull and lack movement and emotion.

In "The Murders in the Rue Morgue," the horrible murder of an old woman and her daughter is described. Poe introduces murder in a closed room; the arrest of an innocent person; the discovery of new clues missed by the police; Dupin's deductions from witnesses, showing his superiority by inference; the rapid elimination of impossibilities through deduction and what remains must be the solution. The more outré a case appears, the easier it is to solve. Dupin finally deduces that the murders were committed by a large ape. The story is a complete manual of detective theory and practice, and is a mixed type of story, partly intellectual and partly sensational. It was produced as a motion-picture a few years ago.

In "The Purloined Letter," a stolen document is recovered. By psychological reasoning it is deduced that the letter is to be found in the most obvious place, in full view of the casual observer.

In the above three stories, Poe has outlined all the tricks utilized by most writers of detective fiction up to the present.

Poe further develops his technic in "Thou Art the Man," and in this story introduces the innocent bystander who is implicated by the murderer, the trail of false clues laid by the culprit, the *corpus delicti,* and a final solution by the most unexpected person. The narrator obtains the confession.

Poe wrote another mystery, "The Gold Bug." This

tale is often considered to be his best mystery story. Sayers classifies this tale in the romantic and sensational variety. The finding of a cipher leads to the discovery of a hidden treasure. This mark-where-the-shadow-falls-take-three-paces-to-the-east-and-dig story, is full of thrills and mystery and the solution is explained in the last chapter. Such stories in other books are never dull, but are often nonsensical.

After these works Poe, for reasons unknown, gave up writing mystery and detective fiction.

The Genius of Poe. Poe's stories describe fear and horror with an exquisite exactness of touch. Mysteries are constructed and unraveled with extreme dexterity. Poe was also a conscientious literary artist and technician who revised and perfected his work with meticulous care. The following word picture is an excellent forensic description:

The body was quite warm. Upon examining it, many excoriations were perceived, no doubt occasioned by the violence with which it had been thrust up [the chimney]. Upon the face were many severe scratches, and, upon the throat dark bruises, and deep indentations, of finger nails as if the deceased had been throttled to death. . . . The party made its way into a small paved yard in the rear of the building, where lay the corpse of the old lady, with her throat so entirely cut that, upon an attempt to raise her, the head fell off. The body as well as the head, was fearfully mutilated—the former so much so as scarcely to retain any resemblance of humanity.

Let us think of Poe, working by candle-light, neatly writing these descriptions in long-hand, correcting, often revising and re-writing several times, with tireless care, until he has perfected his word picture. As good and accurate a description of the scene of the crime as any modern medical examiner could make, even when supplemented by police photography, measurements, and so forth. He wasted no words, knew where to put the comma and the semicolon.

Compare this with our present-day methods of writing. We now talk into the dictaphone; the typist prepares a double-spaced copy with plenty of margin; it may be read the next day, hurriedly corrected and again talked into the dictaphone. Repeated use of the dictaphone and a good typist finally completes the *magnum opus* in short order. Then, composed of poorly constructed sentences and thoughts, repetitions, unnecessary words,[3] and so on, the material is hastily sent to the editor, just under the dead line. We have almost forgotten the art of writing.

SIR ARTHUR CONAN DOYLE

Conan Doyle was born in 1859. He received his medical degree from Edinburgh University in 1885. In 1886, he started practice as an ophthalmologist in Southsea, a small English sea-side resort. Practice was poor and Doyle began to write to keep himself oc-

---

[3] The use of unnecessary words, always reminds me of the story of the fish-monger who had a sign out "Fresh Fish for Sale here." Said his critic, "The word *fresh* is unnecessary, you would not sell stale fish; *for sale* is redundant, you would not give it away; *here* is not needed, it could not be elsewhere; and the word *fish* is not required since you can smell it for two blocks. Take down the sign."

cupied. In 1887, *A Study in Scarlet* was published. In this story Doyle created his undying character, Sherlock Holmes. This was so well received that the other Sherlock Holmes stories followed in rapid succession: 1889, *The Sign of Four;* 1890, *The Adventures of Sherlock Holmes;* 1893, *The Memoirs of Sherlock Holmes;* 1902, *The Hound of the Baskervilles.* A further demand for Sherlock Holmes stories forced Doyle to bring back his famous character in *The Return of Sherlock Holmes* in 1905. Doyle attained world-wide popularity and in 1902 he was knighted.

In later years Sir Arthur became an ardent spiritualist. This was probably the result of that most terrible of degenerative diseases, hardening of the cerebral arteries. In this condition previously intelligent men begin to cut paper dolls, paste pictures in scrap books, etc. Sir Arthur Conan Doyle died in 1930 at the age of seventy-one.

Sherlock Holmes. The creation of the character Sherlock Holmes, was undoubtedly based upon two facts. While studying medicine Doyle came into close contact with the famous Scotch anatomist and surgeon John Bell. Bell would quiz the student for hours on a single bone. Is the bone from a male or female, how tall, what was his build, what was his general appearance and characteristics, did the deceased limp, was he suffering from any disease, what was his occupation? This experience must have impressed Doyle and I believe it was responsible for many of the uncanny observations and weird deductions made by Sherlock Holmes. Secondly, Doyle must have admired and have been familiar with Poe's stories, since he closely copied, followed, and often improved, the Poe technic.

Sayers states that in Sherlock Holmes, Doyle created an eccentric, private detective or consultant in criminal investigations, modeled closely after Poe's Dupin. Holmes used cocaine instead of candle-light and at odd moments was given to playing the fiddle.

In Holmes, Doyle created a character in literature, the secular equivalent of canonization—a real live character. So real has this character become that at the present time it is a common occurrence to see Holmes and Dr. Watson still used in the advertising of whiskies, in telephone advertisements, and the like.

The late William Gillette's excellent characterization of Sherlock Holmes on the legitimate stage has firmly fixed the appearance, manner, and dress of this character upon the minds of the recent generation. Sidney Paget's famous original drawings for Doyle's first works should be consulted by those whose interest may be stirred.

Dr. Watson. In Dr. Watson, Doyle created an honest, faithful, general practitioner to act as the narrator and stooge. It will be seen later, that in modern criminal investigations the doctor assumes a different and more important rôle.

FROM DOYLE TO THE CONTEMPORARIES

Sayers concludes that Doyle took up the Poe formula and galvanized it into life and popularity. The elaborate, psychological introductions were replaced by crisp dialogue. Doyle developed a sparkling, short, snappy, surprising, conversational style—the triumph of the epigram. He made staggering conclusions and deductions from trifling indications. He enriched literature with more than one memorable aphorism. From Doyle to the present time, the writers of dedective and mystery fiction, have with but few exceptions, followed the technic devised by Poe and perfected by Doyle. It is of interest at this point, to illustrate the types of murder and suicide which actually occur, as well as the manner in which they are portrayed on the screen, on the air, and in contemporaneous mystery fiction.

Methods Used in Actual Murder

The actual mode and technic of murder is quite constant. The methods are not numerous, most of them are quite simple and while many are bloody, they are as a rule not at all sensational. The various types may be classified into simple groups. The common methods employed are clearly shown by a study of the murders occurring in New York City during any one year. The total number is greater than that which occurs in the entire British Isles during a similar period, and is greater than those called to the attention of the Federal Bureau of Investigation in any single year.

TABLE I

MURDERS IN THE CITY OF NEW YORK DURING 1935

Methods Employed, in Order of Frequency		Murders
Shooting		197
Stabbing and cutting		109
Assault (with blunt instruments, fist fights, brawls, etc.)		87
Strangulation, smothering, etc.		13
Infanticide		12
Poison		7
Illuminating gas	5	
Other poisons	2	
Drowning		1

Total number during year		426

(About 3 per cent of the 15,557 cases investigated)

Is is of interest to note how uncommonly poison is employed with homicidal intent. This is fortunate, for though homicide by poisoning involves premeditation and the extreme penalty, it is more difficult to convict for murder by this method than by any other.

Most of the murders in large cities are committed in fights, drunken brawls, and because of jealousy or revenge, and are performed with little or no premeditation. This fact must be considered in any criticism of the small percentage of murderers who receive capital punishment or life imprisonment.

In this country only a small percentage of murderers pay the death penalty, and all use every possible means to defeat justice. Thus, the statistics quoted by either side in any discussion of the value of capital punishment can have little actual value. It is my opinion, however, that the quick apprehension and conviction of murderers who may be required to pay the extreme penalty, is the best known deterrent from organized or promiscuous murder.

The significant feature of our deplorable murder situation is that one-half of all homicides are committed by shooting. The cause of this plight is well known.

Hoffman (1),[4] states:

Firearms in this country are obtainable almost by any one, and they are carried by many regardless of the law on the subject. Detective magazines carry a string of advertisements of cheap revolvers guaranteed to kill. Mail order houses furnish weapons to any one, old or young, sane or insane, good or bad, without the least difficulty. Similar advertisements, even more alluring to the criminal mind, appear in numerous monthlies of large circulation. It may be urged that a large amount of crime in this country calls for a more effective method of self-defense, but any one familiar with present day dangers to innocent parties knows full well that unless a person is trained to shoot to kill on sight, possession of firearms only increases the danger, while it gives the offender a chance to escape punishment on the ground of self-defense. The average unarmed person is much safer in the presence of a criminal than the armed person untrained to shoot to kill.

[4] Numbers in parentheses refer to the References, pages 170-1.

HOW WRITERS OF FICTION MURDER VICTIMS

In fiction, the common, ordinary, garden variety of murder has long since been exhausted. Ordinary manual strangulation no longer creates a sensation and receives but passing notice by the press, unless the victim be a Hollywood luminary. Thus, authors of mystery stories are compelled to seek new and bizarre methods of "bumping off" their characters. It is surprising to note how many of these writers pester medical examiners and toxicologists for new leads.[5]

Some of the unusual murders devised by these writers have been: licking of poisoned stamps, poisoned tooth fillings, poisoned boiled eggs, poisoned fruits and candies, poisoned mattresses, poison gas, shaving brushes infected with anthrax, and hypodermic injections (tetanus, allergens, and the like). Further, knives dropping through ceilings, stabbing with icicles, which soon melt and disappear, exposure to extreme cold, electrocution by the telephone, pouring boiling lead into ears, injection of air in arteries and veins, guns concealed in cameras, explosion of timed bombs, death by frightening, radium poisoning (which takes too long and is not recommended), insulin injections, heavy water, *ad nauseam*.

Almost every conceivable method for taking human life has been postulated. It is of great interest to note

[5] The medicolegal background for many of the "Craig Kennedy" stories was contributed by a New York Coroner's Physician, the late Otto Schultze.

that the new discoveries in medicine, chemistry, physics, and other natural sciences, appear to offer the best suggestions for novel ways of committing murder. However, there are methods of slaying which cannot be detected by our present toxicological methods, or by any other means. For obvious reasons, however, such methods could not be publicized.

DISPOSAL OF THE *CORPUS DELICTI* [6]

Fiction writers, in their enthusiasm, describe bizarre, unusual, and often nonsensical, methods of murder which far outdo those seen in real life. Yet, in the disposal of the dead body, the novelists have not even approached the sheer horror which is actually encountered. Perhaps the dead, putrifying, stinking body is a little too nauseating for the delicate, neurotic stomach.

In detective stories the villain attempts to dispose of the *corpus delicti*, which is so necessary for conviction. This has been done by substituting one corpse for another, by burying in lye, and so forth, always with the idea of destruction beyond recognition. With modern methods of identification and proper medical examination of the remaining parts such methods are usually unsuccessful. Other fanciful and impractical methods such as mummification, electro-

[6] "The body of a crime; the essential facts of a crime." In forensic medicine, the term is applied to the dead body of the victim. In the courts, however, it also includes any evidence which is conclusive of death by foul play, such as bullets, knife blade, clothing worn by deceased, photographs of victim, and so on.

plating, planting of the body on innocent persons, and so forth, have been utilized.

To illustrate the ends to which the murderer will actually go in order to dispose of, or to destroy, the body of his victim, I might cite a few well-known examples of the typical methods employed. I have personally investigated many such cases.

1. *"Taken for a Ride."* Shot and left in stolen automobile or dumped out on road. Occasionally great care is taken to remove all marks of identification from the body and clothing. These cases were more common during the prohibition period in the fights between gangsters and hi-jackers, but this type of murder is still encountered.

2. *"Torch Murders."* The burning of the body beyond recognition, but not always beyond identification:

The Moran Case, 1929

Late one dark night in the Newark meadows, a parked sedan burst into flames. Four men were seen to run from the car, jump into another, and set off at terrific speed in the direction of New York. When the fire was extinguished, the charred remains of a body were found inside the car.

A collection of the skeleton and surrounding ashes after an eighteen-hour autopsy revealed that the victim had been shot in the back of the head, soaked with alcohol, and the body set afire. The lungs contained soot, showing that the victim had inhaled smoke from the fire.

A police bulletin was prepared giving the approximate age, height (which was estimated from measurements of the long bones, since the feet were burned off), weight and build, a description of a stiff left elbow joint, manner of dress (obtained by cleaning the human grease off small bits of clothing found in ashes), size of belt, silk (bootlegger's) shorts, etc., and teeth, giving the character of the dental work, bad or good, how recent, etc. A large reproduction of an X-ray showing a gold-capped molar tooth with gutta-percha root fillings was included, and this bulletin was mailed as "An appeal to all dentists" to more than 20,000 dentists throughout the Eastern and middle parts of the country.

In great secrecy, a dentist finally called at my laboratories with dental films taken during life. These showed the identical gold-capped tooth with its gutta-percha fillings and characteristic bone trabeculæ by which the victim was positively identified.

By this time, two of the murderers had been "rubbed out" in New York, a third was in a gun fight with police but never apprehended, and the fourth, known as "Dimples," finding that the police were on the track of a "moll" of the murdered man, killed her. The woman's body was found some time later in the Harlem River with a wire around her neck.

3. *Mutilation.* A common form of disposal of the body by dismemberment. The parts may be dumped in a river or in other places, and are often scattered over a wide area:

The Ruxton Case, 1935

Mrs. Ruxton, the wife of a physician, and her maid disappeared from their home in Lancaster, England. About two weeks later, forty-five pieces of human remains were found along the banks of a stream in Scotland, 110 miles from the home of Dr. Ruxton. Most of the pieces were wrapped in four bundles composed of newspapers and sheeting. Two heads wrapped in cotton wool, a thigh and two forearms were found near these bundles. Twelve additional pieces of flesh, including a pelvis and forearm, were found a few days later further down the stream.

Very careful study of these parts were made by the Scotch anatomists and medicolegal experts. By painstaking X-ray examinations, accurate measurements compared with measurements made with enlargements of photographs of the missing woman, moulages of the feet which fitted into the shoes of the victims, superimposed photography, etc., they were able to reconstruct two human bodies and make positive identification. Dr. Ruxton was arrested, convicted and hanged.

While the police work in this case was never difficult, the identification of the two bodies is a brilliant example of medicolegal work. The book describing the methods employed should be read by those interested (2).

4. *Burial.* Attempts to dispose of the body by burial in the ground, in cellars, in lye, and so on, are not uncommon:

A New Jersey Case, 1938

A married man was having an affair with another woman. One day his car was found abandoned in the woods. Bloodstains and a bullet hole were found in the car. The man had disappeared, and the woman was also missing. Murder was suspected. For six months the police all over the country were searching for the man and, "believe it or not" he was arrested by a country cop who recognized him from a picture in a cheap detective magazine. He was brought back, confessed to the shooting and led the police to the place of burial in the woods. The body was found in a state of preservation good enough to establish the identity as well as the cause of death.

The Crippen Case, 1910

Fragmentary human remains—internal organs and pieces of flesh, the largest measuring 4x6x12 inches—were found buried under the cellar floor in the London home of Dr. Crippen. No genital organs were found but there were some articles of female clothing and a curler along with a few strands of hair. The doctor's wife had been missing for some time.

Identification of the remains was made from a scar on one of the skin-covered pieces of flesh containing some pubic hairs. Mrs. Crippen was known to have had an abdominal operation many years before.

Crippen was apprehended while attempting to escape to America. He was accompanied by his sweetheart who was dressed as a boy. The captain of the slow steamship on which these two sailed became suspicious and remained in constant communication with Scotland Yard by wireless (the first use of the wireless in capturing criminals). When they landed they were met by an inspector from Scotland Yard who had crossed the ocean on a faster boat. Dr. Crippen was convicted and hanged.

5. *Sack Murders.* A common method of body disposal by gangsters, and others, is to truss the body up in ropes, chains, and so on, or stuff it in a sack,

drop it in the water, or leave it in a barrel, or other places. Sometimes the noose around the victim's neck is put on before death and actual strangulation occurs during struggling:

A New Jersey Case, 1938

A young man, recently married, wife pregnant, alleged that he had been annoyed and threatened by a former sweetheart. One night, while riding in his car, they quarreled, and became so noisy that, to avoid attention, he parked in a lonely spot on the edge of a river close to his place of employment. The fight continued and in a fit of anger he strangled her with his hands, and while she was still alive, tied a clothes-line around her neck and held it tight until she stopped breathing. He then went into his employer's garage, obtained two skid-chains used for heavy duty trucks, trussed up the body, secured the chains with the forty feet of clothes-line (one end of which was already around her neck). With the aid of a hand-truck he moved the body to the end of the dock and dumped it into the river. He continued his daily work the next day as if nothing had happened.

Seventeen days after the murder, the body came to the surface with the sixty pounds of chains. The "floater" was badly distended by the gases of decomposition and the features eaten by crabs. The general description of the body conformed to the record of the missing girl. Her family was sent for and although they could not recognize her, identified the clothing and some jewelry. Positive identification was made from the dental work.

The accused was convicted of second degree murder because there was little or no evidence of premeditation.

In a fit of anger you can strangle your wife by holding her neck a little too long and with the aid of a good lawyer the penalty is rarely more than manslaughter. Some juries on hearing the evidence may even acquit you but you must not tie a rope or a wire around the neck. This shows definite premeditation.

6. *Trunk Murders.* Another gruesome way to dispose of the body is to cram it into a trunk and ship it to various parts of the country.

7. *The Cement Coffin Murders.* What more practical way, and one which might well escape detection, than to conceal the murdered body by throwing it (alive or after death) into a barrel of cement which is later tossed into a river. This method has been recently employed by gangsters.

8. *Camouflaged Murder.* Perhaps the most ingenious, insidious, cunning method of "covering up" murder is to arrange the body and the surroundings in such a manner that suicide or accidental death is suspected. This may so mislead authorities as to require the highest degree of skill and experience in criminal investigation to be able correctly to interpret the findings.

For instance, the murderer may "plant" the gun on the victim. In one of my recent cases, the revolver was planted in the left hand of a right-handed person. Autopsy demonstrated that the course of the bullet in the chest was such that it could have been fired with the right hand but that it was hardly possible to have been fired with the left. A tabloid newspaper wanted to know if we had used the "paraffin test."

This is a much heralded test for the detection of powder grains on the hands of one who has recently fired a revolver. It consists of covering the hand with melted paraffin, peeling this off after setting and pouring a reagent over the cast which yields a blue color with any substance containing nitrates (a small amount of urine on the hands—not an infrequent occurrence—will give the same reaction). Although this test is worthless it has been used in murder trials to demonstrate the extraordinary scientific ability of some of the so-called crime laboratories and their experts. In this connection, some years ago while an expert for the defense, I remember being required to listen to a drug clerk who was little more than a "soda-water jerker," describe the delicate precipitin reactions for the detection of human blood, the technic of which requires a well trained and experienced serologist. This expert quickly withered under cross examination.

Undetected murder has often been committed by taking a drunken victim home, dumping him on his bed and leaving him after quietly turning on the gas. This was the final technic employed in the "bumping off" of "Durable Mike Malloy."

The Malloy Case

Mike Malloy, a "down and out" bum, frequented a tavern in the Bronx. The barkeep and a few of his henchmen, one of whom was an undertaker, carried insurance on Mike, and others as well, whom they had picked to be short lived, either from natural causes, alcohol, accident, or by more subtle means. They "had a racket."

In this case the gang believed that Mike would soon drink himself to death, and they offered him all the whisky he wanted as well as food and shelter, in return for the privilege of paying premiums on Mike's insurance policies in which they were the beneficiaries.

Mike seemed to thrive with regular food and increased amounts of alcohol. Disgusted with their predictions and alarmed at the expense, the gang planned to get rid of Mike. They gave him wood alcohol in his drinks, but Mike liked the taste (some alcoholics have an immunity to the poisonous effects of wood alcohol); they dipped raw oysters in wood alcohol, Mike said they were the best oysters he had ever tasted; they fed him spoiled decaying food, putrifying sardines which they had actually contaminated; they poured water over Mike in midwinter and set him out on a park bench—he never even caught cold; they arranged with a taxi driver to run over him, a broken leg and several months in a hospital resulted, but Mike came back for more. They now grew desperate and after getting Mike drunk, they turned on the gas in his room and left. A doctor, apparently a friend of the gang, signed the death certificate giving the cause of death as lobar pneumonia. The doctor failed to recognize the typical color of the skin in carbon monoxide poisoning and made no attempt to report the death to the medical examiner's office.

The insurance companies suspected this gang and asked for an investigation. The body was exhumed and the autopsy and toxicological examination revealed that death was due to carbon monoxide poisoning. The gang was tried, convicted, and four were electrocuted.

The trouble with most all of the above methods noted and illustrated, is that ingenious as they may be, all eventually fail. Is there then any such thing as the "perfect crime"?

The nearest approach to the apparently perfect murder which I have experienced occurred in 1936. Some boys found the dried and mummified remains of a woman stuffed into two potato sacks. The remains had evidently been tossed from a passing automobile into the underbrush along the edge of a road leading from Atlantic City to Philadelphia. With the aid of all known scientific methods, every effort was made to establish the identity and the cause of death in this case. Neither was successful, the case was a "dud," the investigation a "flop":

Autopsy disclosed the body of a white woman, a two-inch piece of white skin was still recognizable; thirty-five-forty years of age, estimated from the condition of her teeth and from X-rays of her skeleton; 5'2" in height, estimated from measurements of certain long bones and the use of anatomical calculations, for the actual height could not be ascertained due to shrinkage and bending of the body; weight about 115 pounds.

Aside from a pink slip, a wedding ring, the color and texture of the hair still present, and brilliantly painted finger and toe-nails, there were no other marks of identification. Dental identification was of little value on account of the cheap character of the work and the probability that the old extractions had never been charted. Fingerprints were obtainable from two fingers by special technic but there was no record of any such prints having been made during life. A plastic reconstruction of the head was finally made for identification.

The autopsy showed no evidence that death had resulted from shooting, cutting or stabbing, or assault with any blunt instrument. There were no broken bones nor fractured skull. Manual strangulation could not be ascertained due to decomposition.

The internal organs were shrunken and mummified or destroyed by maggots so that no diseased condition could be recognized which might have caused death. The stomach had disappeared. The uterus was missing. Since this organ is one of the last to decompose, its absence might suggest that it had been infected, or aborted.

Chemical examination of the body was negative for poisons. Of course, the volatile poisons, and especially alcohol could not be determined on account of decomposition. Arsenic could have easily been found if present. Carbon monoxide death was excluded by the appearance of the deep muscles of one thigh which was still moist but did not have the characteristic color.

It was our opinion that the body which was found in December had been dead since summer. After death the body was attacked by maggots, the shells of which were found throughout the body. Dehydration and mummification were apparently due to exposure in a dry atmosphere such as that in a bungalow garret. The body had not been buried.

The most unsatisfactory aspect of this case is that if the body is ever identified, and if any arrests are made, we shall never be able to prove murder. This case illustrates the importance of universal fingerprinting. This victim could still have been identified in a few days after the body was found had she been fingerprinted during life.

SUICIDES

The inhalation of illuminating gas is the common method of suicide in most civilized countries because it is accessible, cheap, and supposedly free from pain. Other methods of suicide are undoubtedly dependent upon the notoriety the various modes are given by the press, and the constant variation in the accessibility of poisons—for instance, suicide by drinking carbolic acid, a common method years ago and popularly known as the "Dutch act," is now very unusual. Jumping from buildings, which was previously rare, now ranks third in frequency as a mode of suicide in large cities. Suicides from auto exhaust in individual garages, increases in spite of much publicity given the danger of running gasoline motors in closed places, since the death can easily be camouflaged as accidental and double indemnity may be collected by the mourners. Such deaths are usually suicidal, but are often classified as accidental due to lack of collateral evidence. The curtailing of double indemnity, or the cancellation of insurance in all deaths from carbon monoxide, would reduce the number of such suicides.

Many of the so-called accidental deaths from illuminating gas or drowning, are undoubtedly suicides. The question of suicide often depends almost entirely on the police investigation, history, and collateral evidence collected, and when the evidence is questionable the deceased is usually given the benefit of the doubt. The attempt to conceal suicide by families, or friends, is a constant difficulty with which all medical examiners must contend. For these reasons, no accurate classification of the types and causes of suicide can be made.

In a large number of suicides, the following appear to be the underlying factors: despondency because of financial difficulties, actual hunger, chronic illness or incurable diseases, neglect of the elderly by their families, friends, and communities, the increasing number of those suffering from inferiority complexes and manic depressive psychoses (accounting for an increased suicide rate in the young), disappointments in love, and so on. While the suicide rate undoubtedly fluctuates with various economic depressions, the rate remains high and is normally quite constant. Suicide among the members of the colored race is uncommon and since "relief" is plentiful, such suicides should be rare.

I have been of the opinion that some form of religion is a great deterrent to suicide and in our present generation the general breakdown of morale will undoubtedly result in an increased suicide rate.

To illustrate the common methods used in committing suicide, let us refer to one year's record of New York City:

TABLE II

SUICIDES IN THE CITY OF NEW YORK DURING 1935

Methods Employed, in Order of Frequency		Suicides
Illuminating gas		406
Hanging		246
Jumping		207
From building	174	
From other structures, under trains, etc.	33	
Poisoning		146
Cyanides	36	
Lysol	25	
Bichloride	16	
Hypnotics and narcotics	23	
Carbolic	3	
Other poisons	43	
Shooting		134
Cutting and stabbing		37
Drowning		20
Other methods		14
Total number during year		1,210

(About 8 per cent of 15,557 cases investigated)

Suicide Notes. Only a small number of suicides leave notes. This is unfortunate in one way, since the presence of a suicide note would clear up many doubtful cases.

Since 1925, my office has been collecting suicide notes with the hope that eventually some psychiatric analysis of value may be made from these documents which are so intensely human. However, after examining hundreds of such notes I have concluded that any intelligent layman could probably interpret the cause for suicide as given in these testaments, about as well as a board of specialists.

A few typical suicide notes may illustrate this point with little or no discussion:

1. *Financial Difficulties*

> No eats
> "   money
> "   friends
>   time to go

The placing of the ditto marks should be noted.

2. *Inferiority Complex*

John, excuse me for doing this i cannot stand it any longer every boddy is down on me thirty eight years is along time every Boddy spitting on me goot by your truly

Or more tersely:

> The responsibilities of life are too great

3. *Sickness or Incurable Disease*

> good By all   Grandma

Grandma, old and paralyzed, confined to a cot in the garret. A large family, just surviving the economic situation, unwittingly neglected the old lady. No one came up to see her. They forgot to bring the bedpan, and so on. In disgust, grandma took the "gaspipe." No stronger sermon could be preached to impress upon us a lesson in our conduct towards our parents. Similar instances occur daily in families well able to offer every comfort to the old folks.

4. *Revenge or Spirit of Getting Even*

> I am now free from my wife who is no dam good

Or for the benefit of the ladies:

> John the drunken bum is the cause of it all

5. *Thoughtful and Considerate*

Mamie   There is 10$10 Dollers for the Gas I usid

Or in case of a suicide by drinking a solution of cyanide:

> ... P.S.   Throw the glass and spoon away because they are poisoned, and also throw the poison away

THE FUTURE OF DETECTIVE AND MYSTERY FICTION

It has been held that interest in classical literature is on the wane. Some feel that the fine works, the stand-bys of classical education are soon to be replaced by graphic methods. Martin (3), in humorous vein, concludes that we are living in

a picture world, a Leica-chromo age, and although it still helps somewhat to be able to make out the words under the pictures or in the balloons that come from the mouths in comics and cartoons, it isn't necessary. . . . Less and less is it a useful accomplishment to be able to read and write. The movies, the radio, the television yet to come, can be enjoyed by morons unable to spell "cat." . . . The Chinese say that one picture is worth ten thousand words. . . . One picture may say ten thousand words, but ten thousand pictures cancel out all meaning. . . . On the upper reaches, even the serious thinkers must have their pictographs to make statistics easy, and the museums are using swell new cycloram techniques. Photohistories and photo-novels are beginning to come out. The standard newspapers have not been conquered by the tabloids, but they have survived only by adopting the tab picture methods. All the reader-interest surveys show that more attention is paid to the roto section, the comics, and the news pictures than any other part of the paper. . . . On the newsstand the picture magazines are running amuck. . . . How many millions of subintelligences are still left in this great land of schools and colleges as a market, millions as yet unfed by *Click* and *Life* and *Look,* by *See,* and *Pic,* and *Pix,* and *Picture,* and *Fota,* and *Peek?* The potential market is the whole population, the entire 125,000,000 joblot of us who desert the exacting word en masse for the easy picture.[7]

While the neglect of classical literature may be regrettable in that individuals may lack "cultural background," I am not so sure that this should be regarded as a sign of degeneration or national decay. For, accompanying this lack of interest, we find increased attention paid to the natural sciences, and we find more and more screen and radio programs devoted to medicine, physics, and other scientific subjects, as well as to the arts (which in general appear to be of more wide-spread interest than ever).

Along with the vivid pictorial methods employed to-day, an American language, has been evolved (4). This characteristic tongue is almost uniformly spoken by 125,000,000 people. Many consider our speech as a degenerative form of the original English, yet whenever it comes into competition with English, as in

[7] Quoted from *Coronet* (May, 1938), by permission of the publishers.

Canada or in the Far East, American usage, or mis-usage, tends to prevail. Why should this be true? Probably because all the slang and new words in the American language make it more expressive and more accurate—it is really an improved form. For example, the word "movie" is apparently better than "cinema" since the English are beginning to adopt the former term.

Thus we find that the average American reader has turned from the classics to various forms of descriptive American literature. Good detective stories, however, are rare and much time and money are spent on expensive nonsensical books, and on short mystery stories of cheap character, most of which have only sensational "eye-appeal." Crime and mystery stories are also produced on the screen (Philo Vance, Charlie Chan, Nero Wolfe, and so on), and on the radio (Gang Busters, Famous Trials, and so on). The shoddy detective and mystery magazines, however, often contain vivid and accurate descriptions of actual crimes taken from data furnished by a police official to some "ghost" writer. The moral effect of a steady diet of such literature is highly questionable.

Crime solution seems to hold great attraction. Clubs have been formed for the study of crime detection. "Photocrime puzzles" are published in the newspapers with the problem on one sheet and the solution on the next page or in next week's number. A late form of entertainment is the "Crime-file" story. This is published in folder form containing all of the data in an alleged crime. Included in chronological order are the facts of the murder, typewritten police reports, letters, and such genuine clues as lipsticks, scrawled blotters legible with a mirror, real ticket stubs, checks, gauze found at the scene of the crime, and so on. All this material is bound in the style of a police folder. Strictly speaking this is not a story at all, but a realistic collection of actual material. When the reader believes that he has solved the crime he turns to the last page for the solution.

II

On the Medical Detection of Crime in the United States [8]

Forensic medicine [9] and the scientific detection of crime are, at present, at a very low ebb of efficiency in this country. To substantiate this statement one has but to scan the daily press accounts of examinations performed and inquests held by coroners.

The excellent work of the Federal Bureau of Investigation and some of the police departments of our larger cities are the only redeeming features in our systems of criminal investigation. However, the

[8] A large part of the discussion in this section is from "The Teaching of Forensic Medicine" delivered at the Annual Meeting of the Medical Society of the State of New York, April 28, 1936, and published in the *New York State Journal of Medicine*, September 1, 1936.

[9] Forensic (L. *foren'sis*, pertaining to the forum or market place) pertaining to, or used in, the courts of justice. In England and on the Continent, "forensic medicine" broadly designates medicine as applied to the law, and includes the terms "legal medicine" and "medical jurisprudence" which are more frequently used in this country.

incarceration or execution of a few "Public Enemies No. 1" does little to retard the incidence of crime, and "crime marches on." However, before any constructive recommendations can be offered, one must critically review our present methods of criminal detection.

THE NECESSITY FOR A UNITED FRONT

Miller (5) states:

There is professional leadership in the health campaign, but not in the campaign against crime. Everybody is against disease, but not everybody is united against crime. There is no identity of feeling or thought among the various anti-crime organizations. We need professionally trained people to do the exploration and prevention and we need some realistic thinking on the subject.

Hoover (6) says:

Each year sees 12,000 murders, 46,981 cases of felonious assault, 283,685 burglaries, 779,956 larcenies, and 247,346 automobile thefts. . . . It is a national disgrace that the average murderer serves only four years. . . . Throughout our country, law enforcement has been hampered, hamstrung, and strangled by the blood-caked hands of crime-affiliated politicians. . . . In every large American city, there is attorney after attorney who makes his living by counseling men he knows to be guilty . . . often he plans with them.

In addition to such crimes as stated above we must add the enormous loss of life due to accidents. Much of this loss is due to criminal carelessness. The members of the great American public speed home to get a quick supper of canned goods, to rush to a moron movie, to hear a damnable crooner or political noise maker on the radio, or to speed on our super-highways bent on spending all their savings on a cheap weekend.

During 1937, there were 39,500 people killed and 1,360,000 injured by automobiles. Accidents in the home accounted for 32,500 fatalities during this year and about half of these were caused by falls. Another 18,000 lost their lives in public accidents such as falls, drowning, burns, and so on; and 19,500 died as the result of industrial accidents. These facts clearly demonstrate, that in spite of all our "safety drives," the prevention of such unnecessary deaths is a growing national problem.

Further, another source of crime or criminal negligence is the functioning of the Workmen's Compensation Act, the "compensation racket." We only need mention here silicosis—the latest of God's gifts to chiseling lawyers, compensation boys, and racketeers. In 1935 there were cases pending in this country in which the sum of the damage asked greatly exceeded $50,000,000. Such cases are usually taken by the lawyer on a "50-50" basis, the cost of the experts to be paid by the plaintiff. The results are often deplorable. If a poor workman or his family deserve compensation, they receive almost nothing when the case is settled. Often if he does not deserve compensation he may get gravy, for the case may be settled out of court. During 1932, one lawyer is said to have received $100,000 in fees from supposed silicosis cases, few of which he was required to try in the courtroom.

THE CORONER'S OFFICE IN THE UNITED STATES

The Almost Universal Use of the Coroner's Office in the United States; the Chief Cause of this Disgraceful Condition. The coroner's office in the United States is mainly responsible for this disgraceful low standard of medicolegal jurisprudence. It was adopted from the English coroner's system which has been in practice for hundreds of years. According to Schultz (7), some modern incumbents delight to believe that it was established at the time of Alfred the Great. It is certain that it existed in 1194. Moley (8) states that "the coroner's office is a product of medieval conditions and has changed very slightly in functions during the centuries in which it has existed in England and America." [10]

Herzog (9) in defining the present coroner's office, states that:

When a dead body is found, or when a person dies under suspicious circumstances or suddenly, or without having had a physician in attendance during his illness, or having had a physician only a few minutes before death occurred, in a well-regulated community, some one in authority must take charge of the body and must, or at least should, determine whether the person dies from so-called

[10] Quoted by permission of The Macmillan Company from Raymond Moley, *The Missouri Crime Wave.*

natural causes—that is, from disease—or by murder, suicide or accident. If death was from disease, the person in authority would determine the nature of the disease and whether perhaps some industrial poison was a contributing or exciting cause: if by murder, how the murder was committed, whether by means of pistol or rifle, hatchet or dagger, strangulation or poison: if by accident, what the cause of the accident was. Throughout most of the States of the Union the coroner is the judicial officer whose duty it is to investigate such deaths. Some thirty-five states have this old coroner's system without substantial change, save in a few of them the inquest has been abolished. In four other states the justice of the peace performs the function of the coroner. In three other states the investigating official performs the coroner's duties, acting on the order of the court or of the prosecuting attorney. In four or five states only is a medical officer put in charge of the investigation of the physical cause of such a death and a legal officer in charge of the rest of the inquiry.[11]

The Inquest. Again in defining the coroner's inquest, Herzog (9) states that:

For the purpose of investigation the coroner holds an inquest over the body, summons witnesses, and impanels a jury which should view the body, listen to the evidence, investigate and determine the cause of death, and decide whether the person died from natural causes or not. The jury may even find that the person came to his death at the hands of a certain person whom the coroner is empowered to apprehend and commit to prison. The coroner's jury is selected by the coroners and no one has any

[11] Quoted by permission of The Bobbs-Merrill Company from Alfred W. Herzog, *Medical Jurisprudence*.

right to challenge a juror. Thus it has happened that in cases in which a woman died from abortion or a man from a bullet wound which entered his back, that a packed jury would find the woman died from pneumonia and that the man committed suicide.[12]

I need but quote what a few authorities have thought of this farcical jury of inquisition:

Moley (8) states:

The inquest is, as a general rule, without value in determining the cause and circumstances attending death. Moreover, as it is now conducted it does not possess the first requirements of a judicial proceeding. Verdicts as determined by coroner's inquests are generally wholly inadequate descriptions of the cause of death and in many cases do not comply with legal requirements.[13]

Wallstein (10) in speaking of the coroner's office in New York City before the adoption of the medical examiner system, says:

The system of coroners' juries, both as to law and practice, makes the administration of justice in the coroner's court a scandal and a farce. Coroners' juries can readily be and actually have been packed with friends of defendants before them. In the field of criminal abortion, far from serving to detect crime, the coroner's system has become the agency for shielding defendants and concealing criminality. In connection with abortion cases, coroners have called or failed to call juries as best suited their purposes, have packed juries, have intentionally

12 *Ibid.*
13 Quoted by The Macmillan Company from Raymond Moley, *The Missouri Crime Wave.*

failed to call necessary witnesses or to cause police investigation or to utilize the results of such investigations when made. Where the available facts have fairly indicated that death was due to criminal abortion, coroners have without further investigation attributed death to causes unknown.

Imagine, then, the detection of crime, the arrest of individuals, the necessity for necropsy, and the determination of the cause and manner of death dependent upon the verdict of a jury unschooled in law or medicine and too often woefully lacking in general education or knowledge.

The Incumbent. The efficiency of any system depends mainly upon the type of men employed. In this respect the coroner's system is no exception. It is possible but infrequent to have a good honest coroner's office. When such conditions occur they are handicapped by the limitations of a law which states in effect that they can investigate only cases of known violent death. Some coroner's physicians have actually been sued for investigating a suspected violent death. Herzog (9) states that:

The law as to the rights and duties of the coroner varies in different States of the Union, yet in nearly all States where the office is a political one and only in exceptional cases falls into the hands of a physician who is scientifically trained for medicolegal investigations and takes sufficient interest in the work.[14]

[14] Quoted by permission The Bobbs-Merrill Company from Alfred W. Herzog, *Medical Jurisprudence.*

Wallstein (10), speaking in 1915 of the coroner's office in New York City after consolidation of the greater city up to the time of the medical examiner's act, says:

Of the sixty-five men who have held the office of coroner, not one was thoroughly qualified by training or experience for the adequate performance of his duties. Many of the coroners are absurdly ignorant both as to the legal and the medical aspects of their work. The type of man usually selected to the office of coroner is entirely unfit for the exercise of judicial functions, as shown by the general practice of establishing compromising relations with corporations and others who are frequently involved in litigation before the coroner's court.

It will be seen that the position of coroner usually is held by an individual whose incompetence is matched only by his venality.

Character of Work Performed by Coroner. It is obvious to any one who has studied the subject with an unbiased mind that wherever the coroner's office prevails, ignorance, corruption, and inefficiency is the rule. One has but to follow in the newspapers the crimes handled by coroners to realize that when the coroner enters a case confusion and bungling begin.

Wallstein (10) again states in his survey (1915) of the coroner's office of New York City that:

The elective coroner in New York City represents a combination of power, obscurity, and irresponsibility which has resulted in inefficiency and malfeasance in the administration of the office. With constant temptation and easy opportunity for favoritism and even extortion, with utter lack of supervision and control, and without the slightest preparation and training to create in the coroner's mind a scientific and professional interest in the performance of his duties, the present system could not be better devised intentionally to render improbable, if not impossible, the honest and efficient performance of the important public function entrusted to his office. Civil rights and liabilities have been profoundly affected by the findings of the coroner, whose action in many cases has been a travesty on justice. Coroners have abused their powers to compel the employment of favored undertakers by the unfortunate families of deceased persons. Attempts have not infrequently been made to extort sums of money from insurance companies in return for findings in the companies interest. Most of the coroner's physicians in New York City have been drawn from the ranks of medical mediocrity.[15] The character of their medical examinations may be judged from the fact that the keeper of the morgue testified that they often merely look at the head of the body and that an examination lasting five minutes was an infrequent occurrence. The incompetent medical work of the coroner's physicians persists in the investigation of criminal deaths and deprives the community of an absolutely necessary deterrent to crime. Numerous homicides have undoubtedly failed of detection by reason of this fact. So far as the activity of the coroner's office in New York City is concerned, infanticide and skilful poisoning can be carried on almost with impunity. In the

[15] In fact what saved the face of this office for years was the magnificent work of the late Otto Schultze, a coroner's physician for many years and one who unceasingly worked for a medical examiner system.

most important criminal trials, coroner's physicians frequently testify only from memory. The present coroner's system cannot be continued in this city except as a public scandal and disgrace. It should be abolished immediately. In order to obtain effective performance of the work which the coroner's office should do, the district attorneys of New York and Kings Counties have organized homicide bureaus in their own offices. These bureaus make complete and independent investigations in each case. Through long experience, they have come to pay practically no attention to the coroner's investigations, findings, or conclusions. On the contrary, the district attorney's investigations are sometimes impeded by the bungling interference of the coroner.

Adler (11), in a survey of the condition in Cleveland in 1921, states that:

Indeed, we cannot entirely suppress a sense of the ridiculous when we read over the list of causes of death as officially recorded by the coroner of Cuyahoga County for the year 1919.

Consider from the point of view of law enforcement and the public safety, such records as these:

No. 22964: Found dead
22987: Found dead in shanty
22990: Head severed from body
23035: Could be assault or diabetes
23050: Premature or abortion
23187: Diabetes, tuberculosis or nervous indigestion
23484: Found crushed
23551: Died suddenly after taking medicine
23574: Body entirely burned

23686: Shock
23687: Body covered with sores

As a result of public opinion and the work of a Citizen's Committee the coroner's office was abolished in 1915 in New York City, but there was enough political influence to prevent the medical examiner system from going into effect until 1917.

Dr. Norris (the first chief medical examiner of New York City) often told the story that during the days of the coroner's office in New York City, when the coroner and his physician were paid by the piece for work done, they would pull a body out of the East River, one coroner and his physician would examine the body on the dock at East 26th Street and sign the required certificate; if business was dull, the morgue keeper would throw the body back into the river with rope attached, and a short time afterward pull it out again and notify another coroner and his physician, this procedure often being repeated over and over.

In summary, the following opinions apply to most coroner's offices in this country:

Du Vivier (12) states that:

A dispassionate study of the office leads one to the inevitable conclusion that it is an institution of government wholly unsuited to the needs of the present day. It is obviously expensive and clearly inefficient. In some cases it is positively dangerous to thus entrust untrained men with important work. In a word, I know of no better illustration of the saying of Goethe that "Nothing is more terrible than active ignorance." The coroner does nothing that must not be done over again. No reliance can be placed on anything he has done nor can he be trusted to do anything right. Every case in which there may be criminal responsibility must be watched. The body of the deceased is barely cold before the experienced prosecutor begins to guard against the probable mistakes of the coroner—the shifting of the furniture of the scene of the crime, the unskilled handling of witnesses, the insufficient identification of the body at the necropsy, the careless identification of the bullet, or knife, or poison, or the clothes worn by the deceased, the danger of newspaper publicity, the observance of the technical requirements of an antemortem statement, the injury from unguarded and unrestricted cross-examination of the people's witnesses, and the many dangers in every homicide case of importance.

Leary (13) concludes that:

This country inherited the coroner system through the colonial and provincial laws that were adopted into its judicial system on the founding of the United States. Under the primitive conditions that existed before police and judicial systems were developed, the coroner and his jury fulfilled a useful purpose. When a death arose from violence two basic questions had to be considered: 1. What caused the death? This could be answered only by medical investigation. 2. Who caused the death? This was a matter for the police and the courts to determine. In answering these questions the coroner was called on to straddle the functions of two professions, medicine and law. Moreover, the antiquated machinery which he governed, creaking with age, operated so slowly that modern police and judicial systems made its findings ineffective and his efforts unnecessary. Under modern conditions the coroner is literally a fifth wheel on the judicial coach, and an unnecessary expense. The controversy concerning the coroner system that has been going on in England during the last few years is the inevitable protest of progress against an anachronism. Antiques belong in museums and should not continue to be parts of the government of every day modern life. The compromise report of a royal committee appointed to correct faults in the coroner system has met with the disapproval of the British Medical Association, as was to be expected.[16]

THE EFFECT OF THE INEFFICIENT CORONER'S OFFICE

The disastrous results of the widespread use of the system of coroner's offices in this country are reflected in the attitude of the public and the medical profession.

Attitude of the Public. Coroner's physicians and medical examiners and those performing the medicolegal autopsy are looked down upon as politicians and not as leaders in their profession.

Since the funds and equipment for this work are furnished by the state, and since there can be no outside financial support, and since this office carries little political patronage, the importance of the coroner's office has been slighted, and the budgets and allowances have been so very low that the position will not attract or maintain a high-class man.

In such localities where graft exists, and they were

16 Quoted by permission of the publishers of the *Journal of the American Medical Association.*

and still are plentiful, the positions are often held by the lowest type of ward-heeling politician, who employs doctors of the lowest medical and social type. Of course, it must be stated that there are competent coroners and coroner's physicians, but they are all too few.

Under this system it is almost impossible to obtain funds or endowments to maintain special research along with and in connection with this work of such a practical nature and of such practical value, because of the fact that this agency for the actual preservation and protection of human life is so closely associated with a political system under which the appointees are usually men of mediocre ability. Even under the medical examiner's system, the preparation of scientific exhibits for the education of the profession and the laity, the publication of scientific works, and so forth, are for the most part financed by moneys taken from the poor pockets of the medical examiner himself.

The great foundations might well feel, and I am told that some of them are beginning to see, the importance and the possibility of endowing medicolegal institutes in large and responsible cities. Millions of dollars are now spent on research which brings far less immediate results than medicolegal research which could prevent and reduce the waste of useful human life.

Attitude of the Medical Profession. For years the medical profession has had not the slightest interest in the medicolegal autopsy and forensic medicine.

Except for a few lectures in medical ethics to enable students to pass their state boards this subject has not been taught. There have been, therefore, no chairs of forensic medicine in this country until recently when such positions were established at Harvard, New York University, and lately by other progressive institutions. The literature to which the student may turn is limited and there have been no successful journals devoted to forensic medicine.

The main reason for this lack of interest shown by the members of the medical profession has been the realization that if they studied and took special training to fit them for this type of work as a life's career, there would be no future for them, since the politician would rarely appoint qualified men. This fact should be remembered, for when any of our public systems collapse there is always a flattering tendency to blame the medical profession if it has been at all involved.

The medical profession is, however, by no means blameless. Professors of pathology in this country have with few exceptions been experimental pathologists and not morbid anatomists. They have seldom been interested in medicolegal pathology.

It should be realized that medicolegal autopsies must of necessity be more thorough than permission autopsies, since official determination of the cause of death allows the examination of the head, cervical spine, organs of mouth, neck, and so on, much of which is prohibited in permission cases. Consequently much material of great educational value to the medical profession is daily observed by medical examiners. Unless this material is used to further our knowledge, much invaluable information is lost.

THE CONTINENTAL SYSTEM

In continental Europe no such office as that of coroner exists. In Austria, Germany, France, Italy, Russia, and the Scandinavian countries, forensic medicine and the scientific detection of crime has reached a high degree of efficiency. In these countries the daily application and utilization of the medical and other sciences in the administration of justice are brought about through organizations known as "Institutes of Legal Medicine." According to Schultz (14), such institutes are an integral part of the ministry of justice, and since the State controls education they are also a part of the university system.

Housing. Such institutes are usually housed in separate buildings, connected with or adjacent to the large municipal hospitals and consequently near the greatest activity and source of material. From an architectural standpoint alone, many are magnificent, dignified, and with splendid working quarters. They are equipped with everything required. For instance, many of the necropsy rooms have provision for Röntgen-ray examination of the cadaver, an equipment practically never seen in necropsy rooms in this country.

Staff. The director is usually a pathologist of renown and professor of forensic medicine at the university. He has permanent tenure of office and carries with him the social respect and rank due university professors. His staff is likewise connected with the university in various capacities.

Main function. The main function, of course, is the detection of crime. The accurate viewing of the body at the scene of death followed by the necropsy to establish the exact cause of death require medical work of the highest order. For this work such institutions are equipped with adequate morgue accommodations, facilities for the recovery, identification, and preservation of bodies, excellent necropsy rooms, laboratories of pathological anatomy and histology, laboratories of chemistry and toxicology, laboratories of bacteriology, serology, and immunology, proper photographic equipment, and museums and libraries of legal medicine. By its close connection with the medical school and other departments of the university, the institute may request aid from any of the departments of the natural sciences, especially physics and general microscopy. In Austria and Germany, for example, experts are nearly always taken from the teaching staff of the medical schools, and provisions are made that the professors of the medical colleges as well as the professors of chemistry shall be called as experts when necessary.

In Austria not only observation of the body but a necropsy is demanded in every case in which there is a possibility of criminality. In both Austria and Germany detailed rules prescribe under what circumstances and in which manner necropsies shall be performed.

Subsidiary Functions. In some localities, in addition to the main functions of these institutes, the various departments of psychiatry, abnormal psychology and delinquency, and criminal anthropology under the guidance of the institute, may furnish the courts with unbiased testimony in cases where this type of expert testimony is necessary.

Laboratory of Police Science. Closely associated with the institutes of legal medicine, and often in the same buildings, are the laboratories of police science. These laboratories deal with the application of scientific methods and facts in the detection and solving of crime, and in the identification and apprehension of criminals, suspects, and important witnesses. They evaluate and preserve circumstantial evidence and utilize fundamental medical sciences and all other natural sciences which may in any way aid in fixing criminal liability.

Results. The main result of the continental system is that it allows the daily application of medical sciences to the needs of the law and justice by highly trained experts in an impartial and better manner than under any other system yet devised.

The advantages to the institutes with a university connection are that the staff of the institute is given university rank and permanent tenure of office, and that forensic medicine is placed on a dignified university level. Opportunity is afforded for research, and publications may be made under the auspices of the university.

The advantages to the university are: the assurance of proper undergraduate teaching of medical jurisprudence by means of practical demonstrations under the guidance of experts; a great increase in pathological material becomes available for teaching and research, especially affording opportunity for the study of lesions and diseases not usually encountered in hospitals, such as sudden deaths, occupational poisonings, and the like; and finally, graduate teaching and training of medicolegal experts becomes possible.

While it may be true that on the continent, the physical equipment of the institutes makes for the finest work in the performance of a complete medicolegal autopsy, it is said that at many of the larger institutes there is laxity in enforcing the requirement that medical experts view the body at the site of crime. However, experience has shown that in many instances a careful analysis of details at the scene of the crime by the medical officers in conjunction with the police, is more important even than the actual necropsy. The late Dr. Norris insisted upon this important feature in the administration of his office, and the Medical Examiners Act specifically requires that a medical officer observe and take charge of the body at the scene of the crime.

THE MEDICAL EXAMINER'S SYSTEM IS SIMILAR TO BUT
IN MANY RESPECTS BETTER THAN THE
CONTINENTAL SYSTEM

The medical examiner system as practiced in New York City and in Essex County (Newark), New Jersey, approaches the efficient continental method and in some respects is more efficient. The office of coroner was abolished in Massachusetts in 1877 and the medical examiner's system introduced. The law passed at that time has remained unchanged in its essential features. Although the medical examiner's system of Massachusetts has been recommended as a model for communities wishing to abolish the coroner's system, it does not compare with that used in New York City and in Essex County, New Jersey.

Massachusetts System. In Massachusetts the medical examiners are appointed by the governor, who selects "able and discreet men learned in the science of medicine" for terms of seven years. Their investigations are limited to "dead bodies of such persons only as are supposed to have come to their death by violence." They are allowed to perform necropsies only "upon being authorized in writing by the district attorney, mayor, or selectmen of the district." Inquests must be held on all railroad accidents and the district or attorney general may direct an inquest to be held in the case of any other casualty, if he so deems necessary. Herzog (15) states that under this law the district attorney or attorney general has practically all the rights which the coroners held heretofore, except that the medical examiners, or "coroner's physicians," as they were called under the coroner's system, are appointed by the governor instead of the coroner. Furthermore, while the medical examiners in Suffolk County (Boston) have been skilled pathologists, those in other parts of Massachusetts are general practitioners of medicine. While the system in Massachusetts is a great deal better than the old coroner's system, it still is far from perfect, if the whole state is judged not by Suffolk County alone but by the average of the rest of the state.

New York City System. While the medical examiner's system was adopted for New York City in 1915, the first chief medical examiner was not appointed until January 1, 1918, the delay being due to the political ravings of the deposed coroners. The law states that "there is hereby established the office of chief medical examiner of the City of New York. The head of the office shall be called chief medical examiner. He shall be appointed from the classified civil service list and be a doctor of medicine and a skilled pathologist and microscopist." The office is, therefore, appointive under civil service, the tenure being indefinite and removal possible only by the municipal civil service after trial upon charges filed by the mayor.

The requirements are such as to forbid the appointment of some mediocre political physician. The law states that candidates must have a degree of M.D. from an approved institution of recognized standing, they must be skilled pathologists, learned in the field of legal medicine, both with regard to the literature and the present state of that science. They must present satisfactory evidence of having done, in an official connection, at least ten years' work in the pathological laboratory of a recognized medical school, hospital, asylum, or public morgue, or in other corresponding official capacity, and of having performed at least five hundred necropsies. They must possess a theoretical or critical knowledge of bacteriology and toxicology, sufficient to enable them to appraise intelligently the work of expert deputies. It is useless for persons who have not had at least this experience to apply for examination. Candidates are required to submit with their applications copies of their publications.

All deaths by violence, sudden deaths, and deaths under circumstances where crime may be suspected, must be reported to the chief medical examiner. After the report, he must "go to dead body and take charge of some." Therefore, until the medical examiner has completed his examination, no one, not even the police, may take charge of or remove the body or any object whatsoever. Neither the police nor the district attorney have any right to interfere with his actions. Whenever in the opinion of the medical examiner a necropsy is required, it may be done. He does not need to wait for any jury of inquest or for written permission from the district attorney. No inquests are held in New York City under this system, the judicial functions now being held before magistrates in the homicide courts and by the grand jury under the guidance of the district attorney, or before a referee in compensation cases.

Essex County, New Jersey System. In 1927 the medical examiner system was adopted in Essex County, in which Newark is situated. It was copied from and is almost the identical replica of the New York office.

Summary. Since the main advantage of the medical examiner's system over that of the coroner's system is the increased ability to determine the exact cause of death by necropsy, we may sum up the situation, as follows:

In the United States, wherever the coroner's system is still in existence, the coroner's physician performs a necropsy whenever the coroner and his jury so directs; in Massachusetts, where the medical examiner system is in force, the medical examiner performs a necropsy whenever so directed by the district attorney, the mayor, or the selectmen (of course, the district attorney usually gives the medical examiner verbal blanket permission to go ahead, but if for any reason coöperation ceases, the medical examiner is legally powerless); while in New York City and Essex County the medical examiners are given full charge of any body to which death has come suddenly, by violence or under suspicious circumstances. They may investigate the death in any way they see fit, being absolutely unhampered, and may perform necropsies whenever they deem it necessary.

The medical examiner's system in New York City and in Essex County are the two outstanding agencies of their kind in the country. It is safe to say that they are the only American systems which compare with the highly efficient continental system. Those cities under the coroner's system can only be compared to the system existing in England, which is notoriously inefficient, being saved only by the low crime incidence due to the inbred English characteristic of obedience to the law and order, and the covering of important crimes by a senior officer of Scotland Yard of such prominence as Sir Bernard Spillsbury.

Schultz (16), in a summary of this law, states that:

The New Jersey law follows in its general provisions that of New York City. The medical examiner, although empowered to administer oaths and examine witnesses, is relieved of one of the worst features of most coroner's laws, namely, coroner's jury, by a paragraph that provides that the medical examiner shall take over the duties previously performed by the coroner but that the "chief medical examiner shall not be required to summon a jury of inquisition." Inquisitional duties usually assigned to the coroner belong properly to the prosecutor's office or to the police departments, where the New Jersey law places them. The New Jersey law might well be used as a model by other States that may awake to the fact that the coroner's office is an inefficient anachronism.

Authority for Necropsy. A bad feature of most laws relating to the coroner is that such laws fail to define clearly the authority of this official in cases that must be referred to him, but in which, after investigation, he can find no reason to suspect violence.

The right or duty of the coroner to perform a necropsy does not seem to be clearly established. He is also subject to civil suit. (In a recent case in New York State, a coroner's physician investigated and autopsied a man found dead with extensive wounds of the head, and he was later sued in the civil courts for performing an autopsy and for causing the relatives of the deceased to suffer severe "mental anguish.")

The New Jersey law briefly but clearly defines the authority to perform autopsy as follows:

If the cause of such death shall by examination be established to the satisfaction of the medical examiner in charge, he shall file a report thereof in the office of the chief medical examiner. If, however, in the opinion of such medical examiner, an autopsy is necessary, the same shall be performed by the chief or assistant medical examiner.

These two short, concise sentences, the first defining the type of cases that shall be reported to the medical examiner and the second authority to perform a necropsy when necessary, form two legs of the tripod which supports the whole medical examiner's system. The third leg represents the type of man that is selected as chief medical examiner. It represents the authority which at once places the medical examiner system above that of the coroner's system in efficiency and usefulness to the public welfare.

Any comparison between the two systems must obviously take into consideration New York City, with a population of over 6,000,000, using the modern medical examiner system and Chicago, the second city of the country, with a population of about 4,000,-000, still using the ancient coroner's system.

It may be roughly stated that about 20 per cent of the total number of deaths occurring in New York City and in Essex County are referred to the medical examiners, while in Chicago less than 10 per cent are referred to the coroner. Furthermore, of the cases referred to the medical examiners, only about 50 per cent are deaths due to violence (homicide, suicide, and casualties). Over 50 per cent of the cases investigated represent non-violent deaths. In Chicago, however, over 93 per cent of the cases referred to the coroner are violent deaths and only 5 per cent due to natural causes. In other words, there are some 10 per cent of the total deaths in Chicago, which under the New York and New Jersey Acts would be reported to the medical examiner, which are never reported to the coroner. In this group murder, poisoning, criminal abortions, and what not, can easily escape detection.

The physicians of Chicago have long recognized the deficiencies of the Cook County Coroner's Office, as have the local press, but not the politician. In 1933, the Institute of Medicine of Chicago issued a brochure for distribution, some of which reads, as follows:

An office established in the twelfth century to serve the interests of the crown or one established to serve the interests of the public of the present time; the incumbents usually selected by election, or appointed by the Governor or Civil Service Commission; the qualifications being none in most States, or physicians who are graduates of accredited medical schools, with special training in pathology; the duties of the office to be two-fold, a medical one to determine causes of death and a legal one to hold damnable inquests (which must be repeated by the State's Attorney if he must prosecute), or a medical duty only, the legal investigations being made by the District or State's Attorney; do you want the work to be done poorly, because of unqualified incumbents, antiquated laws, political influences, or all of these, or to have the work done excellently because of qualified incumbents and clearly defined up-to-date legislative enactments. Which gives the taxpayer more for his money, better safeguards the interests of society, makes for better administration of criminal justice? The nature of the work performed covers the investigation of deaths due to suspected criminal homicide, in which criminal prosecution may follow; investigation of deaths due to suicide and casualty, which may give rise to claims for accident, disability, or life insurance, or for workmen's compensation; investigation of sudden deaths unattended by a physician, to exclude crime and to authorize legal death certificate.

Can the Coroner's Office Be Improved? The efficiency of the medical examiners' system has been proven in the few parts of this country where it actually functions. The police, the courts, the press, and the public, have all given this system the greatest support. Even the stage and the movies now portray the modern "medical examiner" rather than the "coroner." The medical examiner's office, in certain localities, has been so firmly established that politicians hardly dare to interfere. For the most part in this country, however, the investigation of violent deaths is under the jurisdiction of a coroner's system.

It is encouraging to note, that many of the larger cities realize the inefficiency of the coroner's office and are attempting either to abolish or improve existing conditions. In the last few years, the higher-type coroner and coroner's physician, realizing that they must either improve their system or see it abolished, are making a serious and worthy effort to raise it to a higher plane of efficiency (by education of the personnel, and so on). This is being attempted through the national body—the National Association of Coroners. Such efforts reflect a healthy attitude and should be encouraged, for to abolish this system entirely, would in most localities require a referendum vote.

If the efforts to better the coroner's system are really sincere, and if it is desired really to accomplish something, I would first suggest the abolishment of the coroner's inquest (a damnable, unnecessary, and silly affair). Secondly, the law should be revised so that the coroner's physician will have authority to investigate not only violent deaths, but also sudden or suspicious deaths as well. In the latter there often lurks an unsuspected crime. Finally, if there must be a coroner, relegate him to the position of clerk or secretary or superintendent of buildings, so that the authority of proper crime investigation and performance of the medicolegal autopsy can be placed in the hands of trained physicians.

III

On the Medical Detection of Crime and the Development of New York City as a Center for the Teaching of Forensic Medicine

In the medical detection of crime, the physician must play a more important rôle than that of Dr. Watson, who was but a stooge and narrator. Dr. Watson has been transformed into a *medical examiner*. Likewise Sherlock Holmes, the private detective and crime consultant, is now replaced by the various bureaus of police investigation, such as the Detective Bureau, the Bureau of Identification and Missing Persons, the Homicide Squads, experts in ballistics, finger- and foot-printing experts, photographers, and the like.

The private detective fades out of the picture and exists mainly for the investigation of evidence of adultery in dirty divorce cases, strike-breaking, and so on. Many mysteries are now solved at the autopsy table, rather than in the cozy library of Philo Vance.

The official police bureaus working in close association with the medical examiner, constitute the modern team required for the *scientific detection of crime*. Both of these "arms of the law" are important, and must function without friction or jealousy. Such team-work is well exemplified in the activities of the medical examiner's systems as they function in New York City and Essex County, New Jersey. All the following material is based entirely upon the experiences of the medical examiner's offices in these two areas.

THE WORK OF THE MEDICAL EXAMINER

One-fifth of all Deaths Are Responsible to the Medical Examiner. In those two districts which function under the Medical Examiner's law, one-fifth of all the deaths must be investigated by legalized authority in order to determine when, where, how, and by what means, death occurred. Few realize the enormous amount of work this necessitates, or the need for rapid and practical handling of these investigations, twenty-four hours a day, every day of the week, Sundays and holidays not excepted: "Death takes no holiday."

In New York City there are 80,000 deaths each year. Of these, about 15,000 must be investigated by the Medical Examiner's Office to determine the exact cause of death, and the following table illustrates the groups into which these cases fall.

Violent Deaths. It is generally believed by both the laity and the medical profession that medical examiners only see murders, suicides, and deaths due to accident and trauma and that these cases have very little medical interest. Some professors even consider a study of these cases to be below their dignity, and to be of little use to scientific medicine. I know of no more serious mistake. It may be surprising, therefore, to realize that in a modern medical examiner's system, less than 50 per cent of the total number of cases investigated are violent deaths. The remainder, more than 50 per cent, are due to natural causes, which on account of their suddenness or because of suspicious circumstances require investigation by some legalized authority.

TABLE III

CAUSES OF DEATHS REPORTED TO MEDICAL EXAMINER'S OFFICE
1935

Violent Deaths   *Number*
   Homicides ....   427 or about   3 per cent
   Suicides ....   1,210 or about   8 per cent
   Accidents ....   3,930 or about 25 per cent

Sudden and Suspicious Deaths
   Due to natural causes ....   8,747 or about 56 per cent

Other Deaths
   Abortions ....   100 or about 0.6 per cent
   Stillbirths ....   200 or about 1 per cent

Violent deaths consist, chiefly, of highway accidents, homicides and suicides by cutting, stabbing, shooting, and so forth, and injuries due to falls, burns, industrial accidents, and the like.

Many of these cases come to the attention of physicians during life. The lesions found at autopsy are of great surgical value. Among these are the various types of skull fracture and traumatic cerebral hemorrhage, rupture of solid and hollow viscera, fractures of extremities, ribs, and spine, sudden deaths from pulmonary embolism, and infected wounds of extremities and body. The determination of the exact cause of death, by autopsy, is almost mandatory in most cases, since accurate data must be obtained for criminal, civil, and compensation courts, for the proper detection of crime, or the fixing of criminal negligence, and the administration of justice.

Some idea of the amount of necropsy work performed by medical examiners may be gained from the reports of the New York City office which performs over 3,000 autopsies (population over 6,000,-000), and the Essex County office where more than 800 necropsies are performed a year (population 850,000).

It is astounding to note that in some of the largest medical centers, which carry on extensive research work and teach many students, the autopsy service consists of not more than 300 to 400 cases a year. Many of these necropsies are incomplete. It is obvious then, that a great source of surgical and medical material is neglected or lost.

Murder. About 3 or 4 per cent of the total number of cases reported to the medical examiner are homicides. Homicides by shooting form over one-half of the total number of murders occurring in and around the metropolitan district of New York. Other methods of killing, in order of frequency are: stabbing and cutting, assault, poisoning, and strangulation by ligature and hands. Murder by shooting, cutting, and stabbing form over 70 per cent of all murders.

In every case of murder an autopsy must be performed, and every step taken to ascertain the cause of death, apprehend the murderer and bring him to justice. From the medicolegal angle, the study and analysis of each case must be complete and "airtight."

Suicide. Suicide forms about 8 per cent of the total number of cases reported to the medical examiner. Asphyxiation by means of illuminating gas is the most common method employed:

In New York City during a five-year period (1928-1932), of a total of 7,219 suicides, there were 3,003 by illuminating gas (41 per cent). The number of suicidal asphyxiations from carbon monoxide would be much larger if one included many probable suicides, which, because of reasonable doubt or because of lack of proof, are classified as accidental.

Other methods of suicide in their order of frequency are hanging, jumping from buildings, shooting, poisoning, stabbing, and drowning. Many of these cases require autopsy and careful investigations to exclude crime, criminal negligence, and so on. Yet many can be disposed of (without autopsy), if the history of the case and careful examination of the body and surroundings indicate the obvious cause of death.

Casualties. Deaths caused by injuries in all types of accidents form about 25 per cent of the total number of cases referred to the medical examiner. Of these, the great majority are due to the automobile and falls.

The lack of interest in deaths due to accidents is often quite incomprehensible. There are organized societies for the prevention of tuberculosis, cancer, venereal disease, senility, and the like, but little leadership and no initiative have been shown in the prevention of these injuries which cripple, maim, and kill people—and chiefly those who are of important economic value to the community. The recent work of the National Safety Council in educational drives against accidents in civil life and in industry is of inestimable value. The organization of safety drives, first-aid and preventive measures in many of the larger industrial organizations is to be highly commended.

Under the medical examiner's system the majority of these deaths require careful investigation and exact diagnosis by autopsy in order to fix responsibility and to settle in an equitable manner claims for accident, disability, life insurance, workmen's compensation, and so forth.

Occupational Accidents and Diseases. One of the most important duties of the medical examiner is to prevent waste of human life in industry.

All deaths caused by occupational accidents and all deaths resulting from occupational diseases and industrial poisonings are reportable to the medical examiner. Under the coroner's systems little or no attention is paid to such deaths, especially the industrial diseases and poisonings. The proper investigation of these cases should have the support of all those interested in the health of the working-man,

and in seeing that he obtains adequate and just compensation.

The compensation laws differ in the various states.
In those states in which the law specifically mentions
such occupational diseases as poisoning from lead,
mercury, arsenic, phosphorus, benzol, radium, and
so on, and such diseases as anthrax, caisson disease,
silicosis, and the like, only these are compensable.
This is unjust in some ways in that the hazard of a
new industrial poison is often realized only after
sickness or death has occurred. Many industrial compounds receive wide use and cause considerable
damage before their toxicity has received adequate
investigation.

In other states, so-called blanket compensation laws
cover any disease considered occupational by a board
of experts. In still other states there are no compensation laws whatsoever and workmen are indiscrimi-
nately poisoned and have no recourse to the law.

Deaths Due to Natural Causes. Sudden deaths from
natural causes when in apparent health, when unattended by a physician, deaths within twenty-four
hours after admission to a hospital or institution, and
deaths in any unusual or suspicious manner, are reportable to the medical examiner. Such deaths com-
prise slightly more than one-half of all the deaths
investigated by the medical examiner's office. Heart
disease is the predominating cause of death due to
natural causes.

These cases often can be signed out (i.e., the death
certificate is issued) after a careful history and in-

vestigation, but many require careful autopsy and often extensive toxicological examinations to exclude crime and to establish a definite cause of death.

Few are more fitted to discuss sudden death than experienced medical examiners. Daily, he sees actual cases of sudden death, those which occur on the street, while at work, in public places, factories, at home without medical attention, and those dead on arrival at hospitals (DOA'S).

The majority of sudden deaths occur after forty-five years of age (the summit of cardiovascular life), while sudden death in the age group from ten to thirty-five is unusual. It is an interesting fact that over 80 per cent of these deaths occur in males, and illustrates the detrimental effect of exposure, worry (business men), and hard physical work (especially in syphilitic heart disease).

Heart Disease as a Cause of Sudden Death. In a study of 2,000 autopsies of persons who have died suddenly, I have been able accurately to classify the causes of death into groups which may be of great practical value. Based upon this data, it may be stated that in every 10 cases of sudden death, in which there is no evidence of violence or obvious poisoning, the following causes of death may be anticipated: Seven die as the result of organic heart disease—of which five are due to arteriosclerotic heart disease (hardening of the coronary arteries, high blood-pressure and their sequellæ), one to old, acquired syphilis affecting the heart and aorta; and one caused by the old lesions of rheumatic heart disease. One dies from some disease of the nervous system—the ordinary apoplexy not usually causing sudden death. One dies from some disease of the lungs—the alcoholic walking around with pneumonia usually predominates. And, one from a great variety of chronic diseases in which sudden death may at times occur: cirrhosis of liver, pulmonary tuberculosis, and so on.

If we include, not only heart disease, but also cerebral and other hemorrhages, it may be stated that over 90 per cent of sudden deaths are caused by lesions in the cardiovascular system (heart, arteries, arterioles, capillaries, and veins).

The question arises, are any of these deaths preventable, and what relation do they have to over-eating, persistent driving of a tired body, over-play, hurry, anxiety, intense emotions such as anger, fright, worry, and so forth. No one has greater material and better opportunity to study such deaths than the medical examiner and it is hoped that one day this will be recognized, and research and educational facilities will be placed in close connection with the office of the medical examiner.

A MEDICAL EXAMINER'S PHILOSOPHY

It would be indeed unusual if the medical examiner, who daily comes into contact with all manner of death, did not acquire a pessimistic philosophy of life. This is particularly true in regard to "longevity and the mystery of life" about which we hear so much bunk.

I object to the popular belief that medical science or any other science can prolong the span of human life. We must consider ourselves lucky if we live the allotted three score and ten. Sadly, most of us that do survive are not worth very much. Each species appears to have its fixed measure of years, and it is highly doubtful that science has added a day to the biological span of man. It is too much to expect after but one century of scientific endeavor.

Science and especially the medical sciences, however, have accomplished the very important work of enabling more people to live longer *within the normal span*. The great advance in the control of disease allows a greater number of people to reach that period of life in which degenerative lesions prevail (cancer, arteriosclerosis, and the like). This is also the explanation of the high mortality from the cardiovascular diseases. These facts belittle neither medicine nor science, both have magnificent records.

If we conclude then that our years be numbered, a happier life is certainly the reward of a fine code of morals, whether based upon religion or ethics.

WHAT CAUSED DEATH AND DOES CRIME OR CRIMINAL NEGLIGENCE EXIST?

The primary function of the medical examiner is to answer this question, and all other duties of his office are secondary. Any educational system built around such offices, therefore, are *legally* of secondary importance. This fact must never be lost sight of, and this is one reason why it will be difficult—yet not impossible—to develop university teaching around this purely legal authority.

The answer to this question is entirely medical, requiring the highest pathological skill and training, and cannot be properly performed by the ordinary practitioner of medicine or surgery. It involves what is known as the *medical detection of crime*. This consists of the following.

1. Viewing of Body at the Scene of Crime. Every one knows that when a murder is discovered the police are called. Comparatively few know that a member of the medical examiner's staff—all physicians, trained and experienced in the determination of the cause of death—is called simultaneously; and that the law gives him precedence over the police with regard to the body of the victim and its surroundings (17).

In all homicides, suicides, and suspicious deaths, the viewing of the body at the place of death by an experienced medical officer is of vital importance. The medical examiner upon arrival at the scene has precedence over all other individuals and agencies, and until his medical investigation is completed and he has selected and taken possession of such objects as he deems necessary, no one, not even the police, may take charge of or remove the body or any object whatsoever.

Effective coöperation with the police is absolutely essential, and the police and medical examiners work as one unit toward a common cause, namely, the detection of crime and the fixing of criminal negligence.

In suspected murder cases the homicide squads often arrive at the scene before the medical examiner. They are, however, trained to touch nothing until his arrival. Then all work together, the photographer, fingerprint man, and so on. A careful inspection of the body and its surroundings is made noting anything that may assist in determining whether the death was accidental, suicidal, or homicidal. In the event of murder everything which may lead to the detection of the murderer is noted. Proper instruction of the police and ambulance surgeons soon prevents the careless picking up of a weapon if found, or disturbing other important clues.

If there is any doubt as to whether or not the victim is dead, any necessary disturbance of the clothing or moving of the body for resuscitation, and so on, is, of course, permissible.

Notes are made on the spot by the medical examiner, or taken down by his stenographer, describing the position of the body, its temperature, the absence or presence of rigor mortis, how the body is dressed, and the location and description of any obvious wounds. Personal effects and identification cards, letters, and so on, are usually removed at this time by a thorough search of the clothing as this may afford early clues for the police to investigate. After the police photographer has finished the body is sent to the official morgue where it is not undressed or disturbed in any way until the arrival of the medical examiner.

2. *The Medicolegal Autopsy.* A well conducted autopsy is the only reliable and accurate means for determining the exact cause of death. All other methods are, at their best, mere guess work. The performance of a proper medicolegal necropsy requires a wide knowledge of general and special pathological anatomy, and the knowledge of special, technical procedures which may be of great diagnostic importance.

The necropsy is dictated to a stenographer. The celerity and smoothness with which the medical examiner's office can function is of paramount importance. Deaths can be investigated, the exact cause of death determined by necropsy, and the body released, all within a space of a few hours; whereas under the coroner's system, the waiting for a jury, and so forth, may take as long as two days. At the completion of the autopsy such specimens as are needed to further establish the cause of death, or prove the presence of any contributing factor, or for use in identification, are removed. These are examined in the laboratories of the medical examiner.

3. *Laboratories of the Medical Examiner.* Aside from the various examinations of hair, blood, and seminal stains, clothing, powder stains, handwriting, and so on (tests which are usually performed in the police laboratories), it is necessary in a large number of cases for the medical examiner to make microscopic and toxicological examinations of the important organs, or to submit samples of blood and various

body fluids and exudates to bacteriological, chemical, and serological tests.

There must be a distinction, therefore, between the "medical laboratories" and the so-called "crime laboratories" of the police. They must be separately organized, under separate control, but work in perfect accord.

This distinction may not appear at first sight to be important. However, when one realizes that legislators interested in crime may at any time pass loose laws placing all these laboratories together, under a police officer for example, because they do not understand the situation and may consult no one, the importance of stressing the separation of these departments becomes apparent.

Toxicological Laboratories. Next to the actual autopsy, chemistry is most important in the medical detection of crime. Toxicology (the science of poisons) is required in 25 per cent of the autopsies performed by medical examiners to determine the cause of death, or to eliminate contributing factors, particularly alcohol.

Toxicological work is most difficult and entails great responsibility. Every chemist knows how arsenic or strychnine is detected, but to isolate $\frac{1}{250}$th of a grain of strychnine from a mash of liver, kidney, or brain, without losing it; or a drop of alcohol, chloroform or ether from the brain, is an entirely different matter and requires special knowledge, elaborate microchemical technic and constant research which often includes animal experimentation. The person to whom the chemical analysis is entrusted should be a chemist with years of experience in the analysis of necropsy material. He should be accurate and trustworthy. His integrity must be of the highest order and, indeed, above the remotest suspicion because his evidence may be the basis for the acquital of the innocent or the conviction of the guilty.

As a rule most murders and casualties, and many suicides and suspicious deaths (when death is sudden or occurs within a few hours) require chemical analyses to eliminate poison, alcohol, narcotics, and so on.

Since the establishment of the medical examiner's office in New York City in 1918, the toxicologist Dr. Gettler has analyzed over 25,000 human bodies for poison. They analyze annually over 2,000 bodies, not guinea-pigs. This enormous experience, unequaled in quantity, character, and originality in any other city in the world, could never be accomplished in any police laboratory, but only in laboratories connected with large medical centers and universities. It has stamped Gettler as the outstanding toxicologist of the world.

In this office, in all cases of fatal accidents the brain is quantitatively analyzed for alcohol to determine whether alcoholic intoxication was a contributory cause of the accident. It has been our experience that over 20 per cent of all pedestrians killed outright by automobiles are drunk and that alcohol is a contributing factor in 40 per cent of all violent deaths, such as murder, suicide, and accidents of all kinds.

Some of the larger cities have objected to the expense of toxicological work and pay for it piecemeal only when an important poisoning case occurs. No routine toxicological examinations are made.

What occurs in most parts of the country is something like this: A case receives much notoriety in the newspapers. The authorities seek the services of experts who demand exorbitant fees and usually are not experts in this line at all. This condition exists throughout the country at present and was also prevalent in New York City before 1918. The experts in the "Rice Case" (People *v*. Patrick, 1902) cost New York City $30,000 for trying to prove whether death was caused by chloroform or not. No analysis for chloroform was made. Instead they argued it out in court. In our present medical examiner's system a chloroform case of this kind would be completely solved in about two hours by chemical analysis.

Laboratories of Histopathology. A microscopic examination of the important organs is often necessary to establish the cause of death. While most diseases can be recognized at the autopsy by experienced pathologists with the naked eye, a few cannot and require a careful microscopic study to properly interpret the death:

In one of my recent cases, a young man was accused of murdering his helper in an auto truck. Autopsy disclosed practically no cause of death. There was a small abrasion on the scalp probably caused by a fall. Microscopic examination of the heart muscle showed very fine scarring, the result of rheumatic lesions in the coronary arteries.

The cause of death was definitely established by microscopic examination alone as due to old rheumatic heart disease. The accused was freed.

It would be ideal if routine microscopic examinations were made on all autopsies to complete the record as well as for scientific study and research. However, in large offices this has not been possible due to a curtailed budget and lack of technical help.

In addition there are other microscopic studies of great forensic importance. The work carried on for years by Dr. Vance (18) of the New York office, on the "medicolegal examination of hair" has helped solve many murders.

Laboratories of Serology and Bacteriology. Serological examinations are often necessary in the detection of crime, especially in the examination of blood and seminal stains. These include the precipitin tests for the identification of human blood and the use of the blood groups.

Blood grouping is not only used in criminal cases such as murder and rape, for the identification of a certain individual's blood, but are also of forensic use when employed as tests for paternity, in bastardy and false accusation cases.

Simple and elaborate bacteriological tests are sometimes necessary to establish the cause of death. They are most useful in identifying the micro-organism which has caused death in wound infections resulting from various accidents and in criminal abortion cases. Extensive bacteriological examinations must be made in the various types of food poisoning to isolate the organism and properly classify the case.

The medical examiner must have facilities for the performance of this type of work. It can only safely be performed in connection with large hospitals where the investigator is in constant touch with advances in medicine and has the facilities for individual research work.

Natural and Applied Sciences in the Detection of Mysterious Deaths. In addition to the various tests performed in the medical laboratories and the crime laboratories of the police, it may be necessary at times to call on other natural or applied sciences for help in the solving of obscure deaths. In such cases it is especially desirable that medical examiners have university connections, so that they may be able to use the various departments of physics, engineering, and so forth.

An example of the use of physics in determining the cause of mysterious deaths is best illustrated in the cases of the girls who painted watch dials with radium paint:

The Original Radium Cases, 1917-1924

During these years some 800 girls were employed in a factory in New Jersey painting the dials of watches and clocks with luminous paint containing very small amounts of radium. They "pointed" their brushes in their mouths and so swallowed small amounts of radium.

As a result, very small amounts of radium were permanently deposited in their bones, similar to the storage of lead in industrial lead poisoning. But radium, unlike lead, irritates by its continuous radiations. The bones and the blood-forming organs of these girls received millions of tiny "pin-pricks" caused chiefly by alpha bombardment, every second of their lives.

From 1922 to 1924 several of these girls died. Poisoning caused by the swallowing of radium had never been described. No autopsies were performed and the deaths were attributed to a variety of diseases including syphilis.

In 1925, the true nature of these deaths was established by careful autopsy and examination of the bones for radium. It was found that the early cases died as the result of profound anemia and necrosis of the jaw. The bodies contained from 20 to 180 micrograms of radium. Later deaths revealed that girls died as the result of much smaller amounts, even as little as 1 microgram. The difference was that it took longer to kill. Most of these latter girls died from cancer of the bones (sarcoma). To the present there have been more than 20 deaths among the former dial painters from this plant, 12 have died from sarcoma. (A milligram of radium bromide is not much larger than a grain of sand. One microgram is only one-thousandth as large, is invisible, and cannot be detected by any known chemical method. This is interesting when it is recalled that a fatal dose to man of tetanus toxin, one of the most powerful poisons known, is about 1/300 grain.)

Since the amounts of radium in these cases was too small to be detected by chemical tests, all estimations made during life or after death were done by means of electroscopes, electrometers, Geiger counters, gamma-ray detectors, and the like.

IF CRIME EXISTS, WHO CAUSED DEATH?

This is chiefly a matter of apprehension and is entirely the problem of the police and the courts. This work, particularly in the solution of murder, often requires the participation of many branches of the police department: homicide and detective bureaus, police photography at the scene of the crime, fingerprints, footprints, ballistics, moulages, handwriting, identification bureaus, missing persons bureaus, and so on. Further, coöperation of these departments with the prosecutor's office is required for the preparation of the case for indictment and trial.

Much of the laboratory technic involved in these police activities could never be done in the medical laboratories. However, this separation of the medical and police laboratories does not necessarily imply that these laboratories must be housed in separate buildings. On the contrary, the ideal medicolegal institute would have all these facilities under one roof.

THE DEVELOPMENT OF NEW YORK CITY AS A CENTER FOR
THE TEACHING OF FORENSIC MEDICINE

Twenty years ago the Committee on Public Health Relations of the New York Academy of Medicine helped to abolish the coroner's system in the five boroughs of the City of New York. For many years this Committee has advocated the establishment of an Institute of Forensic Medicine in New York, because of the unparalleled opportunities for study of the vast material available at the Chief Medical Examiner's Office in this area. The following is an account of the progress which has been made toward the accomplishment of this end:

Report of National Research Council. In 1932, Schultz (14), in a careful survey of the possibilities and the need for development of legal medicine throughout the United States, refers to the office of Chief Medical Examiner of New York City, as follows:

The office of Chief Medical Examiner of New York City, with the great volume and variety of work that it must undertake, could easily become one of the outstanding agencies of its kind in the world. Everything, except the necessary financial support, is at hand for efficient public service, for the training of experts in legal medicine for service in other parts of the country, and for the development of medicolegal science through practical application, research, and investigation.

Work of the New York Office. The office of the Chief Medical Examiner of New York City in close coöperation with the homicide squads, detective bureau, bureau of missing persons, and the police academy, investigate more medicolegal cases than any similar organization in the world. Because of this fact and the experience and caliber of the personnel, foreign training in legal medicine is no longer necessary. Everything is at hand for efficient public service except the necessary financial support. The amount of work performed by this office is illustrated by the following table:

TABLE IV

OFFICE OF CHIEF MEDICAL EXAMINER OF NEW YORK CITY:
DEATHS INVESTIGATED, 1918-1937

Deaths	Number
Total investigated	300,000
Homicides	8,000
Suicides	26,000
Casualties (accidents of all kinds)	80,000
Sudden and suspicious deaths	160,000

Department of Forensic Medicine at New York University. In January, 1933, a department of forensic medicine was established at New York University College of Medicine with Dr. Charles Norris (first Chief Medical Examiner of New York City), as Professor. Dr. Norris organized a staff of his associates at the Bellevue Hospital, including the toxicologist Gettler, and the author, the medical examiner of Essex County, New Jersey. In 1932 the first endowed chair of legal medicine was created in this country at the Harvard University Medical School. Until recently these two universities were the only ones to maintain departments for the teaching of legal medicine.

Prior to 1933, at New York University, instruction in forensic medicine had only been given to the fourth year medical students. Similar teaching had been carried on by the same members of the staff of the medical examiner's office at other medical schools in New York City. However, with the establishment of the department of forensic medicine, graduate teaching was organized at the New York University Medical College. Short intensive courses were prepared. Longer courses were organized both in legal medicine and in toxicology which lead to the degree of Doctor of Medical Science or a Doctor of Philosophy in Chemistry, after three years' study.

The Letter of the Mayor. In October, 1935, Mayor La Guardia, in a letter to the New York Academy of Medicine, mentioned the recent death of Dr. Norris, and stated that this "left a great gap in the office of the Medical Examiner of the City of New York, as the function and activities of that office were so definitely centered around his unusual personality." The Mayor requested that, under the direction of the Academy, a study should be made as to what might be done to improve the Medical Examiner's Office, to obtain more financial support (since Dr. Norris had personally paid for the work of additional secretaries and technicians in this office), and to organize the enormous material so that it might be used for educational purposes—not only to train men for a career in legal medicine, but to develop practical research which might eventually save thousands of useful lives.

In the realization of the need for properly trained experts in forensic medicine and the proposal to establish an Institute of Forensic Medicine (which would make New York City the outstanding center for legal medicine in the world), Mayor La Guardia has shown breadth of vision and intelligence rarely encountered in public officials.

Report of the New York Academy of Medicine. At the request of Mayor La Guardia, the Committee on Public Health Relations re-studied the work of the Medical Examiner's Office in collaboration with the present Chief Medical Examiner (Dr. Gonzales), the deans of the medical schools in New York City and an advisory committee of experts. Tentative plans for the establishment of an Institute of Forensic Medicine centering about the office of the Chief Medical Examiner were formulated. This was done in such manner as not to interfere with, but actually to safeguard the official responsibilities of the Chief Medical Examiner's office.

An elaborate educational program was planned to cover every field of legal medicine. The faculty of the institute would consist of members of the Chief Medical Examiner's staff, members of the department of forensic medicine of New York University, and the faculty of the various departments of other New York universities and medical colleges.

All who have the interest of the future of forensic medicine in this country at heart, and all who hope for the betterment of the medical detection of crime, should strongly support the establishment of such a proposed institute.

THE TYPE OF MEN REQUIRED IN FORENSIC MEDICINE

In the opinion of Littlejohn, "there is only one path to the mastery of forensic medicine, and that is, an extensive practical experience acquired by a daily

whole-time application and study of the medical problems which are presented by the crimes of a large
community."

Furthermore the best men for such positions must
be intelligent, possess a good background, while not
being so unbending that they cannot understand the
daily problems of the masses. The medical examiner
must have a good training in gross and microscopic
pathology and an adequate knowledge of bacteriology, serology, chemistry, and the natural sciences. He
must be honest, not subject to flattery, kind and simple in his manner. He must be able to see the human
side in order to weigh properly evidence of all kinds
in a logical manner, and realize the limitations of
circumstantial or other evidence.

He must be a ceaseless, tireless, inveterate worker,
ready to give his time and effort without stint. Death
occurs at any hour, any day. The medical examiner's
work is arduous and he must be cool, sober, and well
able to give testimony in simple, straightforward, understandable style. There can be no mistakes here
since the judicial taking of life often depends on his
investigation and testimony.

And above all this is no vocation for a swivel-chair
pathologist, or a writer of library papers, or for a
long-haired professor who requires sabbatical leave in
Cannes, or a haven in a marble-halled institution of
so-called medical research.

REFERENCES

1. HOFFMAN, FREDERICK L.—*The Homicide Problem* (The Prudential Press, 1925).
2. GLAISTER, JOHN, and BRASH, JAMES COUPER.—*Medicolegal Aspects of the Ruxton Case* (William Wood & Company, Baltimore, 1937).
3. MARTIN, LAWRENCE.—"The New Illiteracy: Why read when you can look? and why think when you can buy it in predigested form?" *Coronet,* May, 1938.
4. MENCKEN, H. L.—*The American Language,* 4th Edition (New York, Alfred A. Knopf, 1937).
5. MILLER, JUSTIN.—Public address, 1935.
6. HOOVER, J. EDGAR.—Public address, 1935.
7. SCHULTZ, OSCAR T., and MORGAN, E. M.—"The Coroner and the Medical Examiner," National Research Council Bulletin, No. 64, Washington, D. C., 1928, p. 7.
8. MOLEY, RAYMOND.—"The Sheriff and Coroner," part 2, *The Missouri Crime Wave* (New York, Macmillan, 1926).
9. HERZOG, ALFRED W.—*Medical Jurisprudence* (Indianapolis, Bobbs-Merrill, 1931), p. 5.
10. WALLSTEIN, LEONARD M., Commissioner of Accounts, City of New York: Report on Special Examination of the Accounts and Methods of the Office of Coroner in the City of New York, 1915.
11. ADLER, HERMAN M.—"Medical Science and Criminal Justice," part 5, Cleveland Foundation, Survey of Criminal Justice in Cleveland, 1921.
12. DU VIVIER, JOSEPH.—*The Abolition of the Office of Coroner in New York City* (New York City, The New York Short Ballot Organization, 1914).

13. LEARY, TIMOTHY.—*Journal of the American Medical Association*, 106, 1408, 1936.
14. SCHULTZ, OSCAR T.—Possibilities and Need for Development of Legal Medicine in the United States, National Research Council Bulletin, No. 87, Washington, D. C., 1932, p. 1.
15. See Herzog, Alfred W., *op. cit.*, p. 10.
16. See Schultz, Oscar T., *op. cit.*, p. 36.
17. MARTEN, M. EDWARD.—*The Doctor Looks at Murder* (New York, Doubleday, Doran, 1937).
18. VANCE, B. M., personal communication.

In the preparation of this article the author has quoted parts of the Ninth Ludvig Hektoen Lecture on Recent Progress in the Medicolegal Field in the United States, given by him, February 24, 1933, before the Institute of Medicine, Chicago, Illinois.

IV

MEDICINE IN THE MIDDLE AGES

BY

JAMES J. WALSH, M.D., Ph.D.

EXTENSION PROFESSOR, FORDHAM UNIVERSITY

IV

MEDICINE IN THE MIDDLE AGES

THERE IS an old story that has gone the rounds until one almost hesitates to repeat it. It is about an Irishman—the Irish are not only humorous in themselves but the cause of humor in others—who picked up on a second-hand bookstore bargain counter an old book on natural history. He was surprised to find in the table of contents a title which ran, "Snakes in Ireland." He knew there were no snakes in Ireland and this made him all the more indignant at the title. In high dudgeon he turned over to the page indicated and found that the whole of the chapter on "Snakes in Ireland" consisted of a single brief sentence: "There are no snakes in Ireland."

I am more than a little inclined to think that a great many people are under the persuasion that an authentic discourse on "Medicine in the Middle Ages" should be nearly as brief as that chapter on the snakes in Ireland. At best they consider it would be made up almost entirely of quotations from some old medieval practitioners who knew very little about science and still less about medicine; that there was nothing like genuine medicine in the Middle Ages and what was studied and applied in the medical schools consisted mainly of astrology and of the descriptions of mixtures of various nasty drugs and old-fashioned remedial measures that came into and went out of vogue, meaning very little for humanity except whatever influence they might possibly have upon the minds of patients. These were bolstered up with some medical superstitions and incantations, together with a number of suggestions that went with the use of medicine in treatments of various kinds that had no true efficacy though they had a value in mental influence that helped sufferers from various affections to get over their ills as soon as possible.

Let me give an example or two of some of the things that are usually supposed to be typically medieval in medicine and are supposed to indicate how little like anything scientific or truly efficacious was to be found in connection with medieval medicine. The Middle Ages were the Dark Ages, one couldn't expect anything serious from them, and they are interesting mainly because they were so amusing in their readiness to accept all sorts of foolish notions in medical practice.

Here is what would be supposed to be a typical medical scene from the Middle Ages, not one but half a dozen physicians at least being present, and each giving a consultant's opinion which out of courtesy had to be followed. A king of England while shaving fell unconscious in his bedroom. It was probably a case of nephritic coma. The royal physicians met and this is how he was treated:

A pint of blood was extracted from his right arm, then eight ounces from the left shoulder, after that he was given an emetic, and two physics, as well as an enema comprising fifteen different substances. Then his head was shaved, and a blister raised on his scalp. It was hoped thus to relieve whatever was causing the unconsciousness.

Then to purge the brain a sneezing powder was given and cowslip powder to strengthen it. Meanwhile more emetics were given and soothing drinks and the royal patient was bled again. Also a plaster of pitch and pigeon dung was applied to the royal feet. Not to leave anything undone, the following substances were taken internally: melon seeds (as a youngster I was once given these though I do not remember what for), manna (which used to be in the pharmacopœia until recently), slippery elm (which I had administered to me to overcome a persistent cough), black cherry water, extract of lily-of-the-valley, peony, lavender (which I remember being used around the house), pearls dissolved in vinegar, gentian root, nutmeg, and finally, forty drops of extract of human skull.

In spite of all this the patient did not get well. As a last resort pills of bezoar stone were employed. The bezoar stone formed in the stomachs of ruminant animals and was supposed to be a very valuable substance for the treatment of all sorts of internal and external ills. It failed in this case. The royal patient died. How easy it would be to say, and how complete a critique of the treatment it would seem, that the poor physicians could not be better than their times, and in the Middle Ages what else might be expected than to get something of this kind? The story comes from MacKinney's book, *Early Medieval Medicine,* and the patient was Charles II, King of England, but Charles II, instead of being medieval in any sense of the word, is quite modern. He died about 1685. That would be nearly two hundred and fifty years after the end of the Middle Ages. So don't blame the Middle Ages for this. It is very modern. It was at this time that the Royal Society was founded in England and Charles himself was a very prominent factor in its foundation. It was he who propounded the famous question to his fellow members: "Why does a pail of water with a live fish in it weigh no more than if the fish were not present?"—a question I leave to the reader to debate.

It is extremely interesting to note the time of origin of a great many things in medicine that are supposed to be medieval and are so proclaimed frequently by people who ought to know much better. These often prove on careful investigation to represent improperly dated historical material or supposed origins that are without authentification.

To repeat another story. Some years ago, more years than I care to mention, an enterprising young chap who wanted very much to study medicine but whose parents could not afford to send him to medical school, took up employment in a drug-store, as they so often did during the nineteenth century in lieu of pre-medical training as we have it. He thought that he would at least get a practical introduction to drugs in this way and become familiar with them, perhaps learn how to treat the simpler diseases, and

in general secure an introduction to medicine such as
would surely be valuable to him in the practice of his
profession later on in life.

He was an observant young fellow, as his subsequent career demonstrated very clearly, and he very
soon had it impressed upon him that one of the most
important medicines so far as frequency of sales was
concerned was one called the theriac. It was surprising how popular it was. People came in to the chemist
shop, sometimes from long distances in the country,
bringing their own bottles with them and asking
that they be filled up with the theriac. The boy clerk
was given the privilege of filling up these bottles
from a large jug in the cellar and collecting the tariff
for them. People who came to buy were enthusiastic
about the value of the theriac as an almost universal
medicine in the sense of doing good for nearly every
ailment under the sun and a good many others besides. The customers confided to the boy how much
of benefit they and their families derived from it.
Many of the old women patients told him that they
would not for the world be without a bottle of the
theriac in the house. It was surprising, the boy
thought, how much confidence the buyers had in this
wonderful remedy. He had no hint of its composition, but one of the steps in progress that he looked
forward confidently to as his term of service continued was that, besides selling the theriac, he would
have the privilege of knowing the secret of its composition as well as compounding this remedy of which
more was sold than any other that they had in the

store. It looked as though this secret would be the most valuable bit of knowledge that he could acquire as a foundation for his practice of medicine. As we have said, it was almost a universal curative agent.

After a time he was taken aside and the secret of the theriac was confided to him. It was an easy compound to make. Whenever any drug spoiled on the shelves it was dumped into the theriac jug which was kept in the cellar. Whenever a drug threw down a precipitate, or when it stained the inside of a bottle indicating that some change in composition had taken place, it was poured into the theriac jug. Whenever a drug clerk, in making up a prescription, made a mistake as to the quantity of the drug needed in the compound he disposed of it by pouring it into the theriac jug. Whenever a drug had too offensive a smell, or whenever it developed a smell if it had not had one at the beginning, it was dumped into the theriac jug. One thing was sure about the composition, that at one time or another it had nearly every drug in the store in its composition.

It was a very great disappointment to the young drug clerk, so excited at the thought that the mystery of the medicine was to be revealed to him, to find that it was only a harbor for mistakes of various kinds, a refuge for many pharmacologic sins, and nothing more.

In the midst of his disappointment which might easily, it would seem, have diverted him from his purpose of studying medicine with the high ideals of helpfulness for humanity which he had cultivated, this young fellow vowed that if it were at all possible he would make such studies in the administration of drugs as would make this sort of thing—the use of the multi-ingredient theriac—hereafter impossible. And he did so, for the young fellow to whom that happened was Claude Bernard, a distinguished French physiologist, who began that fruitful study of the glands of internal secretion that has done more to revolutionize medicine than any other set of discoveries, except those of Pasteur, in the history of modern medicine. The boy had dispensed the theriac and heard the praise of it, but now there was to be no more of things of that kind if his studies could only be made successful. That sounds like an experience straight out of the heart of the Middle Ages.

So far as the theriac itself was concerned, it came from very old times. Galen seems to have used it, but there are hints of its having been used even before that. Galen lived in Marcus Aurelius' time, toward the end of the second century after Christ, but the Alexandrian tradition of medicine has more than a hint of the theriac. In the old times the theriac consisted of a large number of drugs, indeed it consisted of so many that it was spoken of as a calendar prescription, as if it had as many drugs in its composition as there were days in the month, or a gunshot prescription so that if one medicine in it would not cure, another would, and if one affection would not yield to certain of the drugs, it surely would to others. Claude Bernard's story of the theriac as he saw it in his drugstore practice took place about the middle of the nineteenth century. We have a picture of some twenty centuries before us, then, with the theriac in nearly all of them. They used it during the Middle Ages, oh, yes, liberally and fearlessly, but they used it the same way about the middle of the nineteenth century, and they had used it some two thousand years before that. The theriac is in medieval medicine, but it is also in ancient and modern medicine. If the student of the history of medicine learns to date his data, it will be surprising how little originates in the Middle Ages though the Middle Ages accepted many remedies and modes of treatment from antiquity and passed them on to the Renaissance and then to modern medicine, especially passing over some of the most absurd medical ideas to be found anywhere in the history of medicine.

Meticulous care in the study of original sources in the history of the Middle Ages has changed most of our ideas with regard to this period. The general conviction has been that the Middle Ages were the dark ages and that for a thousand years men were sunk in ignorance and utter incapacity to accomplish anything of importance. As the French say, we have changed all that, and changed it all so notably that the period looks quite different now from what it did even at the end of the nineteenth century. The writer of the "Preface" of the *Cambridge Modern History* summed that up very well at the beginning of this generation. He said: "Great additions have of late been made to our knowledge of the past. The long conspiracy against the revelation of truth has gradually given way, and competing historians all over the civilized world have been zealous to take advantage of the change. The printing of archives has kept pace with the admission of inquiry, and the total mass of new matter which the last half century has accumulated amounts to many thousands of volumes." [1]

When Professor Lynn Thorndike of Columbia set forth how much research would be needed before we could consider our studies to be anything like adequate for the period, it was a distinct surprise to those who felt that we must be making great progress in learning about the past. His suggestion was that to make the thousands of manuscripts as yet unedited in the various libraries of Europe and the archives of governments available for students of history, some two hundred years at least would be needed. There is a famous work in Europe, that of the bollandists, which comprises the lives of all the saints, at which scholarly men have been working for two hundred and fifty years and they expect that it will take at least a hundred years more to complete. That is the way we look forward now to accretions of knowledge with regard to the Middle Ages. We no longer think of them as the Dark Ages.

Our own John Fiske said of them: "When we think of all the work big with promise of the future that went on in those centuries which modern writers in their ignorance used to set apart and stigmatize

[1] *Cambridge Modern History,* Editor, A. W. Ward (New York, The Macmillan Company, 1912). Quoted by permission of the publisher.

as the dark ages, when we consider how the seeds of what is noblest in modern life were then painfully sown on the soil which imperial Rome had prepared ... there is a sense in which the most brilliant achievements of pagan antiquity are dwarfed in comparison with these." [2]

John Fiske would be inclined to put these Middle Ages ahead even of the brilliant achievements of pagan antiquity. He adds: "Until quite lately indeed the student of history has had his attention too narrowly confined to the ages that have been preëminent in literature and art—the so-called classical ages—and thus the sense of historical perspective has been impaired." [3]

What we have found is that these men of the Middle Ages built the great Gothic cathedrals which have remained ever since a triumph of architectural engineering and construction work that has become the favorite subject of study for our architectural students of the modern time. The word Gothic came to be applied to them because they had been built by our rude Gothic ancestors (so the Renaissance people said) who knew no better, but see what a change has taken place. Now every town in America of a hundred thousand inhabitants has a Gothic church in it and our larger cities have Gothic cathedrals but none of them can vie for beauty with the great Gothic

[2] *The Beginnings of New England or the Puritan Theocracy in Its Relations to Civil and Religious Liberty* (Cambridge, The Riverside Press, 1889), p. 18. (Boston, Houghton Mifflin Company), Quoted by permission of the publisher.
[3] *Ibid.*

churches of England and France built in the despised Middle Ages.

In connection with the cathedrals came the foundation of the universities. Canons of the cathedrals were the first group of teachers in the universities. During the Middle Ages literally many thousands of students flocked to these universities. The basis of the university teaching was the seven liberal arts, which Huxley declared to be better calculated to develop the many-sided mind of man than the curriculum of any modern university. Some years ago I found that all the colonial colleges, seven in number —Harvard, William and Mary, Princeton, Pennsylvania, King's College (now Columbia), Yale, and Brown—followed this scholastic teaching, as the programs for their commencement exercises demonstrated very clearly. We had deprecated Scholasticism while all the time our colleges were following very closely in the footsteps of the medieval colleges even including the disputations which it has been the custom in recent years to discredit, though the reason why the Declaration of Independence and the Constitution of the United States are so thoroughly conservative is exactly because of the sound training of mind received in those old Colonial colleges.

DIAGNOSIS

Most people would be very much inclined to think that medieval physicians occupied themselves almost exclusively with treatment and paid comparatively little attention to diagnosis, that is, the recognition and differentiation of one disease from another. According to them, the diagnostic side of medicine would be presumed to exist mainly in glittering generalities and diagnosis would be in very general terms. All states of fever would be called fever, and if any particular organ gave symptoms then the word fever and the organ were combined in order to describe the disease. It is true that many affections were described in terms of the various humors, four of which were particularly emphasized—blood, bile, lymph, and phlegm. But curiously enough more attention is being paid to these humors now than for several generations and there is a distinct tendency to a recognition of the fact that the humors of the body, deeply influenced in constitution as they are by the secretion from the endocrine glands, have a great deal more to do with at least the indirect causation of diseases of various kinds than has been thought down to very recent years.

As a matter of fact, it is surprising to find how many diagnostic terms that are used very commonly at the present time were also in use during the Middle Ages. Bartholomew the Englishman, as he is called, in his book on medicine in the encyclopedia which he wrote under the title *The Properties of Things,* gives a great many of these terms for symptoms and suggests their significance and also their treatment. He begins with the head and goes down through the body, calling attention to the various affections to which the parts of the body may be subjected. Perhaps the best way to illustrate how modern many of Bartholomew's terms are is to name over some of them with brief comments. One of his earliest chapters—they are really rather long paragraphs—is with regard to headache. He begins by describing migraine, says that it is due to fumes from the stomach, the symptoms of which are, as it were, a beating of hammers, and the patient cannot bear noise nor the slightest disturbance, nor light nor shining. He describes the headache also that comes with a pricking and burning sensation, and with running from the eyes and from the nose. He is evidently describing what we call hay fever or certain symptom complexes resembling it.

Another capitulum is on catarrh, or running from the head. He describes a summer and a winter catarrh. The one is a common cold, and the other a summer catarrh in which "great superfluity cometh out at the nose and at the mouth." Two paragraphs later he describes the causes of and remedies for delirium or frenzy which he attributes to the head, and then he has a capitulum on vertigo, and one on wakefulness, the familiar insomnia, and then one on the falling sickness or epilepsy. He has no less than six capitula on affections of the eyes. Among them he describes sub-conjunctival hemorrhage, and involuntary tears, chronic inflammation of the tear sac. He discusses both defective vision, and blindness or privation of vision, and suggests certain remedies. He then takes up deafness and its causes, its connection with dizziness and gives suggestions for the treatment. Remember that all this is in a volume that was published before the middle of the thirteenth century. Among the diseases of the nose he has a capitulum or brief chapter on polyps in connection with fetor of the nose which we call ozena.

Perhaps the most surprising capitulum in Bartholomew's book on medicine is his description and treatment of a symptom complex for which a nice long Greek name has become familiar in recent years as a result of an intensive advertising campaign that caught everybody's attention. Bartholomew called it fetor of the mouth but it has become popularized in recent years as halitosis.

Bartholomew has the following to say about this affection. The quote is from the English edition of 1495, a time when they were very frank in their mode of expressing what they wanted to say. It would not, I imagine, be nearly so frankly discussed nowadays if the old-fashioned English terms for it were used. Bartholomew says:

Stinking of the mouth comes sometimes from corruption of the teeth and of the gums, and sometimes of sores and pimples of the palate and of the mouth. Sometimes it is due to an affection of the chest. Sometimes it comes from rotted (that is putrefied) humors of the stomach. Sometimes it comes from universal and entire affection of the body as happens in lepers. Sometimes mouth fetor comes from the eating of stinking things, as happens in the case of those who are always eating garlic, onions and leeks.

This affection can be cured with cleansing and sweet

smelling and strengthening medicines. In this case the matter in the stomach is the cause of the stink, and it must be dissolved and broken up and put out. Often after eating, spewing [that is, vomiting] must be excited, and thus the chambers of the stomach be cleansed and purged. The patient must beware and avoid foods that are disposed to putrefaction and he shall use sweet smelling wine to strengthen him.

If the bad breath come from some other cause, as of rotted teeth, or from the gums, these teeth that are the cause shall be drawn out and the gums shall be rubbed and cleansed with a decoction of roses in wine or they shall be washed with lukewarm vinegar. The gums and the roots of the teeth shall be rubbed and cleansed with powder of *thus* and with *mastick* and *honey*.

With regard to toothache Bartholomew suggests that milk is a good food for the teeth and he thinks that chewing, that is, vigorous mastication, is extremely important for the preservation of the teeth, and he evidently reached the conclusion to which our dentists are returning, that the diet and the internal humors have more to do with the condition of the teeth than the conditions within the mouth. He talks of the bluntness of teeth in old age and had evidently seen a number of these cases where the teeth are worn down from chewing particularly hard things.

Some of the other capitula that Bartholomew writes are with regard to aphasia, hoarseness, quinsy, and suffocations of the throat, difficulty of respiration as to inspiration and expiration, purulent or bloody sputum, consumption, palpitation of the heart (Bar-

tholomew calls it "cardiac passion"); and then there
are a number of capitula, nearly a dozen in all, on
fever. He talks of ephemeral fever, as well as simple
fever, and of hectic fever, but also putrid fever, probably pyemia. Then he has quotidian, tertian, quartan,
continued, and acute, fever. He devotes a capitulum
to horripilation or "goose flesh," and also one to
nausea, as well as to boulimia or the canine appetite.
There is a capitulum on hiccough, one on vomiting,
one on pain in the belly or stomach, and one on ileus
or colic. He has separate capitula for dysentery and
for lientery, the affection in which food is passed almost without any digestion.

Then there are such familiar names as dropsy,
jaundice, piles, pain in the kidneys, hernia, lumbago,
arthritis, sciatica, gout, ulcers, pustules, scabies, im-
petigo, and prurigo, treated together, and capitula
on leprosy and on morphea or overgrowth of the edges
of a wound. He has a chapter on snake poisoning but
also one on rabid dog bite and treatment of the bites
of poisonous animals.

He has an extremely interesting capitulum on the
physician and his profession. He insists that the
physician be diligent and busy in things that belong
to the craft of medicine, that is, keep himself up-to-
date. He must understand the complexions, that is,
the temperaments of men, their constitution, and the
compounds both of the humors and of the organs that
occur among men. He must also understand the influence of the seasons, the conditions of the male and
female, and of the age of the patient, for one kind

of medicine is needed in winter and another in summer, one kind at the beginning of a sickness, another at the climax, and still another at the passing thereof, one kind in childhood, and another in youth, and still another in full age, and another in old age; one in the males and another in females; and he needs to know causes and occasions of disease and the symptoms and complications. He insists that a medicine may never be taken securely and with assurance if the cause of the disease is unknown.

There is an old medical proverb which was frequently repeated by Dr. Osler. He attributed the origin of it to Dr. Parry of Bath, but it is much older than that. It runs: "It is much more important to know what sort of patient has a disease than what sort of disease a patient has." Bartholomew would agree very cordially with that and he has much more to say than space will allow quotation for.

Bartholomew would insist on knowledge and ever more knowledge in a physician and he emphasizes the fact that rarely does a single drug relieve symptoms that come from various causes. It is the duty of a good physician to set himself to searching the cause and circumstances of a disease. He should search and seek the cause by sight, by handling and groping, that is, by inspection, palpation, and deeper seeking, as well as by the urine and by the pulse. There is a frontispiece to this book on medicine showing the tiled end of the ward of a hospital in which examinations of various kinds are being made. They were intent on the causes of disease just as far as they could get at them.

Popular medicine presents some very interesting medical documents from the Middle Ages. One of these is what is known as the *Regimen Sanitatis Salernitanum,* the *Code of Health of the School of Salerno,* which for centuries was the most popular medical book in Europe and was not only copied in many manuscripts but issued in hundreds of editions after the invention of printing. It is said to have been compiled by the professors who taught medicine at Salerno during the twelfth and thirteenth centuries. The health advice is in rimed Latin verse. Ordinarily rimed Latin verse is thought of as somewhat macaronic, but the rimed Latin hymns of the Church, especially the *Dies Iræ,* the *Stabat Mater,* and others, are now looked upon as some of the greatest poetry that ever was written. Professor Saintsbury of the University of Edinburgh, the distinguished Scottish critic, has declared these Latin hymns the most wonderful wedding of sense and sound that the world has ever known. The *Regimen* is no such poetry, mainly because its subject is commonplace and could not rise to poetic heights, but it served its purpose of impressing on people's minds truths about health in a way that made them easy to remember.

The *Regimen* was not written for physicians but for the laity. It constituted one of a series of many lectures such as these, or such as are gathered in by Bartholomew the Englishman in his *De proprietatibus rerum.*

The book is dedicated to the King of the English by the faculty of the medical school of Salerno. The translation made into English verse by Professor Ordronaux,[4] begins as follows:

> If thou to health and vigor wouldst attain
> Shun weighty cares, all anger deem profane;
> From heavy suppers and much wine abstain
> Nor trivial count it after pompous fare
> To rise from table and to take the air.
> Shun idle noon day slumber, nor delay
> The urgent calls of nature to obey.
> These rules if thou wilt follow to the end
> Thy life to greater length thou mayst extend.

These lines were easy to commit to memory but that led to many different readings and versions. These medieval hygienists of nearly seven centuries ago believed very much in early rising, the use of cold water, thorough cleansing, exercise in the open air, yet without sudden cooling afterwards. The lines on morning hygiene seem worth while:

> At early dawn when first from bed you rise,
> Wash in cold water both your hands and eyes,
> With brush and comb then cleanse your teeth and hair
> And thus refreshed your limbs outstretch with care.
> Such things restore the weary o'ertasked brain
> And to all parts insure a wholesome gain.
> Fresh from the bath, get warm, rest after food,
> Or walk, as seems most suited to your mood.
> But in whate'er engaged or sport or feat
> Cool not too soon the body when in heat.

4 Philadelphia, Lippincott, 1871.

The tradition with regard to not permitting the body to pass suddenly from heat to cold because of the danger of internal congestion, was particularly emphasized by the Salernitan writers and that is probably why it has continued as a tradition among us.

Down at Salerno they did not believe in noonday sleep though as that is on the latitude of Naples there has always been a tendency to take an afternoon siesta, and even the weight of authority of the *Regimen Sanitatis* was not sufficient to overcome this. The old physicians at the health resort insist that sleep in the afternoon makes one feel more tired than less and counsel not to break the day by a sleep at noontime. They said:

Let noontide sleep be brief or none at all,

and they threatened all sorts of misfortunes that might befall him

Who yields to noontide's drowsy call.

They believed in light suppers and insisted that you should wait until your stomach is surely empty before you put anything else into it. Pure air and sunlight were favorite tonics at Salerno as they have been in the modern time. Taking a hair of the dog that bit you was a maxim of the School of Salerno for the cure of potation headaches. They said:

Art sick from vinous surfeiting at night?
Repeat the dose at morn, 'twill set thee right.

The faculty at Salerno insisted that fresh air and milk and eggs were the best possible treatment for consumption. This tradition had come down from the time of Hippocrates who, it is said, told a young man threatened with consumption to "buy a cow and go up into the mountains." At Salerno they recommended various kinds of milk as well as cow's milk. They considered there were special virtues in each kind of milk. There was goat's, camel's, ass's, and sheep's milk, and the use of these probably had a definite psychological influence. Apparently some patients had been seen with an idiosyncrasy for certain kinds of milk and it was deemed better not to insist on their taking milk which had a tendency to disagree with them. It is surprising how much these rules of health at Salerno anticipate some of our maxims of health in the modern time.

There are certain directions that are given for the cure of particular diseases or symptom complexes, such as hoarseness, catarrh, headaches, fistula in ano, so that there was definite information. Here, for instance, are the directions to be given a patient suffering from rheum or catarrh:

> Fast well and watch. Eat hot your daily fare;
> Work some and breathe a warm and humid air.

The advice continues:

> Of drink be spare; your breath at times suspend—

(that is to say, draw a long breath)

> These things observe if you your cold would end.
> A cold whose ill effects extend as far
> As in the chest is known as a catarrh;

> Bronchitis, if into the throat it flows;
> Coryza, if it reach alone the nose.

At the end of the *Regimen*, after their dedication to England's King, the care of the health is boiled down into two lines:

> Use three physicians still—first Dr. Diet,
> Next Dr. Merryman, and third Dr. Quiet.

Popular medicine would seem to be the phase of medicine that would be least considered and above all least developed in the Middle Ages. We have already seen that the *Regimen Sanitatis Salernitanum*, contains a great many of the health precepts and practices that still continue to be bruited about and that represent popular medicine not at its most ridiculous, as might possibly be expected, but at its most commonsensible. The old physicians liked to put things pithily so that people would readily recall them and be able to use them to decided advantage. The aphorisms of Hippocrates, who is often spoken of as the Father of Medicine, represented the beginning of this form of medicine, but we had many other exemplifications of it, some of them very well done indeed, in the course of the Middle Ages.

After the *Regimen* of Salerno, the best known set of these health aphorisms was that written by Maimonides, the great Jewish physician, the royal physician to Saladin, who is so romantically known in the history of those times. Maimonides wrote a series of letters on dietetics for the son of his patron, Saladin. The young prince seems to have suffered from one of the neurotic conditions that seem to develop in those who have their lives all planned for them and little incentive to do things for themselves. The main portion of his complaint centered, as in the case with many another individual of leisure, in disturbances of digestion. Besides, he suffered from constipation and feelings of depression. Most of us would be inclined to think that the son of so great a ruler as Saladin would not suffer from these conventional and almost casual afflictions. Doubtless the young prince, like many another young person, was quite sure that these symptoms portended some insidious organic ailment that would surely bring an early death.

It is very interesting, then, to see what Maimonides gathered together as advice under these circumstances. He begins by insisting on piety, and a healthy mind in a healthy body. He said:

Man is bound to lead a life pleasing to God if he wants to have a healthy body, and he must hold himself far from everything that can hurt his health and accustom himself to whatever renews his strength. He should eat and drink only when hungry and thirsty and should be particularly careful of the regular evacuation of his bowels and of his bladder. He must not delay either of these operations, but as far as possible satisfy the inclination at once.

In his second aphorism Maimonides said:

A man must not overload his stomach but be content always with something less than is necessary to make him feel quite satisfied. He should not drink much during the meal and only of water and wine mixed, taking somewhat more after digestion has begun and after digestion is completed, in moderation according to his needs. Before a man sits down to table he should note whether he has any tendency to evacuation and should make the body warm by movement and activity. After this exercise he should rest a little before taking food. It is very beneficial after work to take a bath and then the meal.

Maimonides gives very specific directions. For instance:

During sleep a man should lie neither on his face nor on his back but on his side, the beginning of the night on his left and at the end on his right. He should not go to sleep for three or four hours after eating and should not sleep during the day.

The old Jewish physician who was undoubtedly the medical genius of that century, said with regard to noxious foods:

There are certain harmful foods that should be avoided. Large salt fish, old cheese, old pickled meat, young new wine, evil-smelling and bitter foods are often poisonous. There are also some which are less harmful, but are not to be recommended as ordinary nutritive materials. Large fish, cheese, milk more than twenty-four hours after milking, the flesh of old oxen, beans, peas, unleavened bread, sauerkraut, onions, radishes and the like. These are to be taken only in small quantities and only in the winter time and they should be avoided in the summer. Beans and lentils are to be recommended neither in winter nor summer.

Meticulously specific directions are given as regards what is good for children and for older people:

Honey and wine are not good for children, though they are beneficial for older people, especially in winter. In summer one-third less of them should be eaten than in winter.

Special care should be taken to have regular movements of the bowels that carry off the impurities of the body. It is an axiom in medicine, that so long as evacuations are absent, or difficult, or require strong efforts, the individual is liable to serious disease. Every medical means should be taken to overcome constipation in order to escape its dangers. For this purpose young people should be given salty food, materials that have been soaked in olive oil, salt itself, or certain vegetable soups with olive oil and salt. Older people should take honey mixed with warm water early in the morning and four hours later should take their breakfast. This proceeding should be followed up from one to four days until the constipation is overcome.

SURGERY

In the eleventh century in the midst of the fermentation set up not only in Europe but also in Asia and Africa in connection with the Crusades, there came into existence down at Naples a medical school which represented the beginning of medical education in Europe. This was at Salerno, which is still a health resort to which people from many parts of the world go because of its salubrious climate. In connection with this health resort which was visited by the nobility and important ecclesiastics from all over the world of that day, there came the establishment of a medical school. The most important teacher in the school was the man who is known as Constantine Africanus, because he was born in Africa. His birthplace was Carthage. He went to school at Kairouen, a Mohammedan city some hundred miles south of Carthage. I visited it some time ago but there are practically no remains of the school there. Kairouen is one of less than half a dozen Mohammedan cities, a visit to which represented the fulfilment of a religious obligation. A visit to Mecca, the home of Mohammed, once, gave assurance of salvation. Three visits to Kairouen gave similar assurance.

What Salerno was famous for proved, surprisingly enough, to be the development of surgery. We are so accustomed to think of surgery as a development of our time that it is rather surprising to find here in the southernmost part of Europe the beginnings of a school of surgery that was famous some eight hundred years ago. Only that we have the books written by the professors of surgery at Salerno would it be impossible to convince anybody in modern times that a series of surgeons made a magnificent beginning of their art some eight centuries ago. Fortunately the books have been preserved for us, they existed in many manuscript copies because the books represented the best surgical practice that was to be found anywhere at that time. Surgery began with a textbook written by two famous surgeons, Roger and Roland

—in Italian, Ruggiero and Rolando—giving us heroic names for the origins in this phase of care for the ailing and the injured. After the textbook of Roger and Roland there came what was known as the book of the Four Masters. Four surgeons independently of one another, apparently, told the story of surgery as it was practised in their time after the distinguished origin of it under Roger and Roland.

Gurlt, the distinguished German historian of surgery, who has written a thoroughly authoritative *History of Surgery,* says that: "In spite of the fact that there is some doubt about the names of the authors, the Four Masters, this volume constitutes one of the most important sources for the history of surgery of the later Middle Ages, and makes it very clear that these writers drew their opinions from a rich experience." It is rather easy to illustrate from the quotations given in Gurlt or from the accounts of their teaching some features of this experience that can scarcely fail to be surprising to modern surgery.

Take the case of fractures of the skull. There were rather emphatic directions not to conclude because the scalp is unbroken that there can be no fracture in the skull. If a man is hit by a metal instrument like the clapper of a bell or by a heavy key or by a rounded instrument made of lead—this would remind one very much of the lead pipe of the modern time, so fruitful of mistakes of diagnosis in head injuries—special care must be taken to look for symptoms in spite of the lack of an external penetrating wound.

These old surgeons knew of the possibility of fracture by contrecoup.[5] They said that, "quite frequently though the percussion comes in the anterior part of the cranium, the cranium is fractured on the opposite side." They even seem to have known of accidents such as we now discuss in connection with the laceration of the middle meningeal artery: "A youth who had a very small wound made by a thrown stone seemed not to be injured seriously but he died the next day. His cranium was opened and a large amount of black blood was found coagulated in the dura mater." Much is said about fractures of the skull. Depressed fractures must be elevated. If the depressed portion is wedged, then an opening should be made with the trephine and an elevating instrument used to relieve pressure. Care should be taken in lifting the skull to protect the soft parts from injury. Gurlt italicizes the expression, "In elevating the cranium be solicitous lest you should infect the dura mater." There are interesting discussions of the prognosis of wounds of the head. If fever develops, the wound is mortal. If the patient loses the use of hands and feet, the wound is mortal. If universal paralysis comes on, the same thing will be true. Operations on the skull must be done where the air can be warmed artificially. Hot plates should surround the patient's head while the operation is being performed. Other means of heating the air near the patient are suggested. Split or crack fractures are diagnosticated by the method of Hippocrates of pouring some colored fluid over the

[5] Injury resulting from a blow on a remote part.

skull after the bone is exposed when the linear fracture would show by a line of discoloration.

They say that surgeons who in every serious wound of the head had recourse to the trephine must be looked upon as "fools and idiots." These old surgeons emphasize the fact that the surgeon's hands must be clean, he must avoid the taking of food that may corrupt the air, such as onions, leeks, and the like, and in general must keep himself in a state of absolute cleanliness. They did not have the meticulous carefulness of the modern surgeon because they had no knowledge of the reasons for it, but they anticipated our modern surgeons in many principles. This textbook of the Four Masters remains down to the present day a very important contribution to surgery.

Gurlt has many thousands of words in his three volume, large octavo history of surgery, with regard to these south Italian surgeons, but he has even more with regard to the north Italian surgeons—men like Ugo da Lucca, Bruno de Longoburgo, Theodoric, and William of Salicet. It might very well be thought that this group of Italian surgeons would be of little more than antiquarian interest for the modern times. It needs but a little first-hand knowledge of what they have written, however, to show how unjust such an opinion as this would be. These Italian surgeons operated so freely that it becomes quite clear that they must have had some facility for putting their patients under an anesthetic before operating on them. Tom Middleton, the English poet contemporary of Shakespeare, in his play, says: "We shall imitate the pities of old surgeons who put their patients to sleep before they cut them." We have a record of the use of an anæsthetic consisting of opium, hyoscyamus, mandrake, and wild lettuce, which they used for the purpose of producing the narcosis. It was not as good as our anæsthesia, though it must not be forgotten that we are still experimenting in the hope of improving our anæsthetic methods; it was not so efficacious, some patients did not stand it as well as others, but it served its purpose.

Another anticipation of modern surgery was antiseptics. I know a good many people will be inclined to say that only somebody very enthusiastically intent on making the Middle Ages anticipate all our modern advance would dare to suggest that medieval surgeons developed not only anæsthesia but also antisepsis. When Professor Clifford Allbutt, Regius Professor of Medicine at the University of Cambridge, England, made his address before the St. Louis World's Fair Congress of Arts and Science at the beginning of this century, he did not hesitate to declare that William of Salicet, the great Italian surgeon of the north of Italy, discussed the causes of union by first intention and the modes by which it might be secured. He too insisted that cleanliness is the most important factor for securing good surgical results.

All of these men insisted on cleanliness as the most important factor for good results in operating upon septic cases. Their wounds were dressed with wine and then linen dressings were steeped in strong wine and placed over the wound. This evaporated, carrying away in the evaporation the germs though, of course, these old surgeons knew nothing of that but must have suspected their existence, and they succeeded in getting union by first intention and boasted of the fact that their wounds healed with linear scars so that they could scarcely be seen. They warned that there was more danger from wounds being infected, that is, not healing well, in summer than in winter. The end of the wound was to remain open in order that lint might be placed thereon to draw off any objectionable material. The preferable suture material Bruno said, according to his experience, was silk or linen. He was particularly insistent on the necessity for drainage. In deep wounds special provision must be made to secure this, but in wounds of the extremities the limb must be so placed as to encourage drainage.

Altogether Gurlt in his *History of Surgery* gives about fifteen large octavo pages of rather small type to what he calls a brief compendium of Bruno's teaching. The other north Italian surgeons are just as famous as those we have mentioned, and for any one who reads German readily, especially if he can also read some Latin, there is abundant material to demonstrate beyond all doubt that surgery with anæsthesia and antisepsis finely developed reached a monumental position in the world of that time.

After the Italian surgeons came the French, most of whom had been taught by the Italians. The first of these great teachers was Lanfranc who was expelled from Italy for political reasons—but then we have had lots of experience with that—and the Visconti proved as harsh dictators as any of our moderns. Lanfranc went to Paris to teach and Gurlt declares he attracted an almost incredible number of scholars to his lessons in Paris, and by hundreds they accompanied him to the bedside of his patients and attended his operations. The dean of the medical faculty urged him to write a textbook of surgery not only for the benefit of his students at Paris but for the sake of the prestige this would confer on the medical school. Many times since deans of medical schools have urged this, and it has proved excellent for the school as well as for the professor and his pupils.

Lanfranc describes the qualities a surgeon should possess. He should have well-formed hands, long slender fingers, a strong body, he should be of deep intelligence, and of a simple, humble, brave, but not audacious, disposition. He should be well grounded in natural science, he should know not only medicine but every part of philosophy, he should know logic well so as to be able to understand what is urged, to talk properly, and to support what he has to say by good reasoning. He deems it well for the surgeon to have spent some time teaching grammar and dialectics and rhetoric, for this practice will add greatly to his teaching power. Some of his expressions might well be repeated in the modern time to young surgeons: "The surgeon should not love difficult cases, and should not allow himself to undertake those that are desperate. He should help the poor as far as he can, but he should not hesitate to ask for good fees from the rich."

It would seem as though they had to face some of the problems that we have at the present time with regard to how the surgeons should give the poor as good treatment as they give to the rich. Our problems are not different from those of the long ago.

Next to Lanfranc in importance is Mondeville who succeeded as professor of surgery at Paris. Mondeville's favorite principle was that there was nothing perfect in things human and successive generations of younger men often made important additions to what their ancestors had left them. He seems to have introduced into practice the idea of the use of a large magnet in order to extract portions of iron from the tissue. He repeats with approval the expression of Avicenna that, "often the confidence of a patient in his physician does more for the cure of a disease than the physician with all his remedies."

Mondeville thought that nursing was extremely important. He considers that nurses must be well trained, faithful, and obedient. He has no use for talkative nurses. He does not hesitate to say that sometimes near relatives are particularly likely to disturb patients. Especially are they prone to let drop some hint of bad news. He thought that wives made particularly poor nurses. Mondeville was very much interested in the irregular practice of medicine and surgery and succeeded in making such regulations as prevented quacks and charlatans from practising as freely as before. He was very much surprised that well-informed people of the better class allowed themselves to be influenced by these quacks. He was surprised also that so many who were not physicians or surgeons presumed to give advice in medical matters. "It thus often happens," he said "that diseases in themselves curable grow to be simple incurable or are made much worse than they were before." He says that some of the clergymen of his time seem to think that a knowledge of medicine is infused into them with the sacrament of Holy Orders.

Another great French surgeon of that time was Guy de Chauliac. He studied for years in Italy and later at the invitation of the pope then residing at Avignon he became the papal physician. He wrote a great textbook of surgery, sometimes spoken of as the greatest surgical work of that time. He died about 1370, his life running concurrently with the years of that century. Chauliac was educated at Montpellier and from there went to Bologna where he attracted the special attention of the leading surgeon of that day, Bertruccio, who was attracting students from all over Europe. Chauliac tells of the methods that Bertruccio used in order that human bodies might be in as good condition as possible for demonstration purposes. He mentions the fact that he saw him do many dissections in different ways.

The great French surgeon's attitude toward anatomy and dissection can be judged from his famous expression that, "the surgeon ignorant of anatomy carves the human body as a blind man carves wood."

How highly he was esteemed will be noted from the fact that he was chamberlain physician to three popes, Clement VI, Innocent VI, and Urban V. He tells us himself that his great textbook, the *Chirurgia Magna,* was undertaken as a *solatium senectutis*—a solace in old age.

Chauliac objected very much to the way that physicians and surgeons followed authority too closely and therefore failed to recognize advances in knowledge. Chauliac said: "While Socrates or Plato may be a friend, truth is a greater friend." His bitterest reproach for many of his predecessors was that "they follow one another like cranes, whether for love or fear I cannot say."

Chauliac's anticipation of modern views in the treatment of abdominal conditions is most surprising. Wounds of the intestine are fatal unless leakage is prevented. He suggested the opening of the abdomen and the sewing up of such intestinal wounds as could be located. Like many another abdominal surgeon he seems even to have invented a special needle holder.

Chauliac describes his method of securing anæsthesia. He says:

Some surgeons prescribe medicaments that send patients to sleep so that the incision may not be felt. For this purpose opium, the juice of the morel, hyoscyamus, mandrake, ivy, hemlock, wild lettuce, are employed. A new sponge is soaked in these juices and left to dry in the sun; and when they have need of it they put this sponge into warm water and then hold it under the nostrils of the patient until he goes to sleep. Then they perform the operation.

Chauliac's own experience seems to have shown that this narcotic could be successfully employed.

INSANE

Very probably the most astonishing feature of the history of medicine in the Middle Ages which has been revealed in recent years is that which concerns the treatment of the insane. The general persuasion is that the insane were treated abominably during the Middle Ages and that, as their condition was considered to be due to possession by evil spirits, a certain amount of moral blame attached to their affection because of which there was very little sympathy for them. They were outcasts, to be manacled and chained for life, if they had shown a tendency to violence at any time. They were fed very badly, they were treated scarcely as human beings, and it is surprising to note man's inhumanity to men and women under the circumstances. Most of this persuasion with regard to medieval treatment of the insane is utterly false.

There is no doubt at all that the insane were very badly treated in the eighteenth and early nineteenth centuries. We hear of Pinel, the distinguished French physician, knocking the shackles off the insane at the end of the eighteenth century, thus creating a distinguished name in humanitarianism in the world of his day. How well I remember the thrill I had on attending some of Pierre Marié's lectures in the very hall in which Pinel knocked off the shackles. Pinel had been preceded, however, in his great good work only a very few years before by the Quakers in England and in this country and by certain philanthropists. It all came as the result of ideas that were fermenting in the minds of men in preparation for the French Revolution, and as a result of this new spirit for the liberty of man which had been introduced into the world at that time.

When we come to the question of the care for the insane during the Middle Ages there is a surprise awaiting people who talk about medieval neglect of the insane and above all the failure to understand that insanity was a disease and was really to be treated as such quite as diseases of the body would be. It is often said that the most frequent cause of insanity as delineated in the Middle Ages was possession by evil spirits. There was comparatively little said about possession by evil spirits during the Middle Ages. The possibility of it was accepted but was not obtrusive. The witchcraft period and the tale of possession by evil spirits had their place in the seventeenth and eighteenth centuries. Probably more than 100,000 people were put to death while the witchcraft delusion was at its height but this was in modern, not medieval, history.

Let me quote a paragraph with regard to the insane and the causes of their affection and the treatment as it comes to us from the Middle Ages. The paragraph is not long, but contains an immense amount of information with regard to the way of looking at the insane which they cultivated in the Middle Ages. Once more the quotation is from our old friend, Bartholomew the Englishman, *Bartolomeus Anglicus* as he is sometimes called. Bartholomew had an interesting background. Two great religious orders, the Dominicans and the Franciscans, were founded in the first quarter of the thirteenth century. A member of the Dominicans, Vincent of Beauvais, became an intimate friend of King Louis IX of France who encouraged him to write an encyclopedia. The size of this can be very well appreciated from the fact that if printed in modern octavo volumes there would be about sixty of them. This was evidently a source of information that could be consulted only in libraries, and the books had to be chained to the shelves in order that the sets might not be broken. I understand that our Public Library in New York loses from their shelves many hundreds of volumes a year. I do not know whether there is question of chains for our books.

The Franciscans were possibly closer to the people than the Dominicans, and so it was proposed to write a smaller encyclopedia in a single volume, containing as much readily available information as possible. This is the well known *De proprietatibus rerum, The Properties of Things,* written by Bartholomew the Franciscan.

His single volume encyclopedia was nearly the size of Webster's unabridged dictionary, as it used to be issued some forty years ago. This encyclopedia was written with the idea that pastors and confessors should have a readily available source of information for answering the questions of their parishioners and penitents. It treated of a great many things in brief capitula or paragraph chapters. One book or division was entirely devoted to medicine, constituting something like one-tenth of the whole work. I have already given you some idea of the medical information in the volume, and now I want to tell you of Bartholomew's attitude toward insanity and how thoroughly he understood it:

Madness cometh sometime of passions of the soul, as of busyness and of great thoughts, of sorrow and of too great study, and of dread; sometime of the biting of a wood [mad] hound, or some other venomous beast; sometime of melancholy meats, and sometime of drink of strong wine. And as the causes be diverse, the tokens and signs be diverse. For some cry and leap and hurt and wound themselves and other men, and darken and hide themselves in privy and secret places. The medicine of them is that they be bound, that they hurt not themselves and other men. And namely, such shall be refreshed, and comforted, and withdrawn from cause and matter of dread and busy thoughts. And they must be gladded with instruments of music, and some deal be occupied.

We still think, with Bartholomew, that madness or insanity comes from passions of the soul, that is, profound emotional disturbances. It comes from overwork, too deep thinking, occurs as a consequence of sorrow, and from overstudy and from dread. He has here all the mental causes of insanity, what might be called the endogenous causes. Now come those from without, the exogenous causes of insanity. It may come from the bite of a mad dog or some other venomous beast. It may come from the eating of melancholy meats. They thought the dark meats ever so much more indigestible in the Middle Ages than we do at the present time. Finally, among the exogenous causes, is the drink of strong wine. Bartholomew evidently knew about alcoholic insanity, and sets it down very succinctly.

And then he says that there are different kinds of insanity. Some of the insane cry and leap and hurt and wound themselves and other men, these are the maniacal; and others darken and hide themselves in privy and secret places, these are the melancholics, the depressive insanity patients. Then comes the treatment. The patients must be bound, that is, not manacled nor chained but so wrapt up and tied in cloths that they hurt not themselves and other men. This was the strait-jacket which is still in use.

Then comes the actual treatment. The patients must be refreshed and comforted. We must get them away from their environment and from whatever causes, dreads, and anxieties, and busy, that is, deeply emotional, thoughts they have. The surprise of the whole situation, however, is in the last line: "The insane must be gladded with instruments of music and some deal be occupied." Here is the occupation and entertainment treatment of the insane which we have been inclined to think that we are the originators of, stated in a very few words in an encyclopedia that was completed sometime before 1250. That encyclopedia is to be found in more manuscript copies than almost any other book except the Bible. When printing came, no less than seventeen editions of Batholomew were issued among the incunabula, that is between 1450 and 1501. Not only did the medieval scholars know the truth about insanity but they expressed it very well and they diffused that information throughout the civilized world of their time.

HOSPITALS

We have come to the erection and the equipment and the construction in detail of what are undoubtedly the finest hospitals in the world. Some of them are lacking in architectural qualities but as hospitals a great many of them are as near perfection as it is possible for them to be. In small as well as large towns the hospitals are often worthy of the progress of medicine and surgery in our day, and they are saving a great many lives and a great deal of suffering.

This is all the more surprising because some of us can recall how much the poor dreaded having to go to hospitals. I can remember it quite well. I was brought up in a mining town about a mile away from an old wooden hospital that always had a good many patients, because besides the folk suffering from the ordinary ills of life, a number of those who were injured in the mines went into the hospital. They did not go, however, if they had any friends. A boarding-house mistress with whom a miner had boarded for a couple of months would feel in duty bound to save him from the hospital if he were ill or injured, and if she did not the community feeling with regard to her was anything but favorable. Hospitals were one degree above poor-houses, and the poor-houses were at that time, the beginning of the fourth quarter of the nineteenth century, about the last place in the world that one would want a relative to go to. The hospitals were not only the dread of the poor but they were real poverty-stricken institutions where only those were treated who had no friends left in the world.

No wonder the poor dreaded hospitals, for the death-rate in them was extremely high. A great many patients who went in for slight ailments or injuries never came out alive. A miner might be admitted for a crushed finger that should be better in the course of a week and allow him to go back to work at the end of a couple of weeks, but instead he came out "feet first," as was the common saying among the people of the neighborhood. This was true not only for the hospitals in small towns but for some of the great hospitals of the world. At the beginning of 1870, Professor Nussbaum, who was the surgical director of the great city hospital in Munich with some 5,000 beds, said: "I will operate in that hospital no more." And no wonder! His operating mortality for the preceding year had been 79 per cent plus, that is to say, four out of five of the patients he operated upon died. That is easy to understand when we realize that Lister's work had not yet affected continental

Europe to any extent, and hospitals reeked with infection. Erysipelas, that scourge of surgery, was nearly always in the wards, various forms of sepsis were nearly always present, septicemia and pyemia were frequently to be seen, and patients died from these infections.

Hospital reform did not come until well on toward the end of the nineteenth century. Many of the most prominent physicians in New York in the last decade of the nineteenth century, were prone to disbelieve the microbic theory of disease and refused utterly to accept the idea of infection for most surgical cases. Surgeons welcomed what they called laudable pus because it was a less virulent form of infection than some of the others, and patients recovered from it. I have seen, while making graduate medical studies in Paris, a distinguished surgeon come into a hospital from his carriage, be ushered immediately into the operating-room, turn up the cuffs of his coat sleeves, dip his hands into a basin of water very daintily, and then proceed to operate. No wonder hospitals got bad records for not saving the lives of many patients.

Once more, as with regard to the use of the theriac, we need to know our dates! During the eighteenth and early nineteenth centuries hospitals were in the worst possible condition. They were quite literally a disgrace to civilization. Their nurses were of a character that the less said about them the better. Dickens in *Martin Chuzzlewit* described Sairey Gamp, and most people are inclined to think that that was a gross caricature while it was, on the contrary, a piece of the most actual realism. It was creatures like the drunken Sairey Gamp who took care of patients in the hospital and it was one of these who said, when the young physician was giving her instructions as to how to care for the women and children in the ward committed to her charge, "Don't you think that I know how to raise children? Haven't I buried six of me own?" When ordinary city hospitals had experiences of this kind, it is easy to understand that the hospitals of poor-houses in country districts represented the veritable limit of inattention to the ailing poor.

If hospitals were as bad as this at the end of the nineteenth and the beginning of the twentieth century, the common feeling would be that they must have been ever so much worse in the early nineteenth century, and they must have been pretty bad in the eighteenth century, and worse, if possible, in the seventeenth, and still worse in the sixteenth century. As for the condition of hospitals in the fifteenth century and earlier, that is, during the Middle Ages, the less said the better. Conditions must have been almost impossible, but the argument does not hold at all. Miss Nutting and Miss Dock in their well known *History of Nursing* call emphatic attention to the fact that a period of decadence in hospital construction, equipment, and organization began just at the end of the Middle Ages and continued to grow worse as time went on until the worst possible hospital conditions existed about the middle of the nineteenth century. Virchow, the great German pathologist, in his article on the history of German hospitals, which is to be found in the second volume of his *Collected Essays on Public Medicine and the History of Epidemics,* tells the story of the foundation of these hospitals, and says that there was a hospital in every town of 5,000 inhabitants in Germany. Those in the larger towns at least were model hospitals in many ways and ever so much better than many hospital structures erected in post-medieval centuries. What was true for Germany was true also for France and for England. The great hospitals of London— St. Thomas's, St. Bartholomew's, Bethlehem (afterwards Bedlam), Bridewell, and Christ's Hospital, the first of which afterwards became a prison, while Christ's Hospital, though retaining its name, became a school—are all foundations made in the thirteenth century. It would be easy to suppose that these hospitals were rather rude structures, inexpertly built, poorly arranged, and above all badly lighted and ventilated. They might be expected to furnish protection from the elements for the poor, but scarcely more. As a matter of fact they were almost exactly the opposite of any such supposition. It is because our generation still has the memory of the hospitals of the past generation and assumes that if these were so bad the hospitals of an earlier time must have been almost impossible that we have the tradition with regard to medieval hospitals that is so unfortunate because it is so far from the truth.

Viollet le Duc in his *Dictionary of Architecture* which, I need scarcely say, is an authority on the subject, has given a picture of the interior of one of these medieval hospitals erected in France by Marguerite of Bourgogne, the sister of King Louis IX. Mr. Arthur Dillon, discussing this hospital from the standpoint of an architect says:

It was an admirable hospital in every way and it is doubtful if we to-day surpass it. It was isolated, the ward was separated from the other buildings, it had the advantages we so often lose of being only one story high, and more space was given each patient than we can now afford.

The ventilation by the great windows and ventilators in the ceiling was excellent. It was cheerfully lighted, and the arrangement of the gallery shielded the patients from dazzling light and from draughts from the windows and afforded an easy means of supervision.

It was, moreover, in great contrast to the cheerless white wards of to-day. The vaulted ceiling was very beautiful; the woodwork was richly carved, and the great windows over the altar were filled with colored glass. Altogether it was one of the best examples of the best period of Gothic architecture.

It was built on the bank of a stream and a small artificial canal carried water around the hospital, and usually infection was not supposed to pass over water.

There was a famous hospital of St. John at Bruges which was erected in the midst of a populous commercial town. Bruges was one of the important cities of Europe at that time. The oldest portion of the hospital provided the most light and air for the patients and the best opportunity for thorough cleansing as well as for occupation of the patients' minds while lying abed. In the hospital of St. John are Memling's famous paintings of St. Ursula and her companions. Memling was an artist who had no money, but was in the hospital for several months and in lieu of money paid his hospital fees with paintings done during convalescence. A small charge is asked for sightseers of these paintings and so many go in to see Memling's paintings that something more than $10,000 a year is collected and the artist is still, nearly five hundred years after his death, paying his hospital fees very bountifully.

PRACTICE

To my mind the most surprising feature of medieval medicine, so far as comparative history is concerned, is the law regulating the practice of medicine which was issued by the Emperor Frederick II just before the middle of the thirteenth century. The law was binding on the two Sicilies, that would be the kingdom of Naples and the island of Sicily, of which Frederick was the ruling monarch. It serves to show exactly the status of medical education seven centuries ago and throws bright light on medical practice in these southern provinces at this time. We are very proud of what we have accomplished in uplifting medical education, in regulating medical practice, and in guaranteeing pure food and drugs during the past generation. Every advance that we think we have made during this time is to be found in this law of Emperor Frederick's.

Before beginning the study of medicine the prospective physician must have studied three years at the seven liberal arts, and especially logic, grammar, and rhetoric, as a definite pre-medical course. In recent years, I believe, it has been felt that a better pre-medical course than one devoted entirely to science is one that offers opportunity for study of the arts and mental development generally rather than confining the mind too soon to scientific subjects.

After this he must devote himself for three years to the study of medicine itself. Then he must practice with a physician for a year before being allowed to take up the practice of medicine on his own account, which corresponds with our year of practical work in a hospital. If he is to take up surgery he must have made during a year special studies in anatomy. This is distinctly laid down in the law in so many words. It is all the more interesting because usually it is said that the study of anatomy was neglected or even forbidden during this century.

One thing more is to be found in the law that is astonishing to say the least under the circumstances. It anticipates by nearly seven centuries our pure drug law which was promulgated only some thirty years ago. All the relations between physician and apothecary are regulated in meticulous fashion so as to make sure that what the physician prescribes shall be dispensed and that the druggist shall always keep fresh, potent drugs on hand and will be in a position to guarantee the medicaments that the physician wants. The enforcement of the law was not left to chance and the penalties inflicted under it were severe and were carried out. The exact wording of the penal clause is: "Violation of this law is to be punished by confiscation of goods and a year in prison for all those who in future dare to practise medicine without such permission from our authority."

We would be prone to wonder what the pre-medical course consisted of, that is, the studies embraced in the curriculum, and we find that these scholars studied what are known as the seven liberal arts, the old trivium and quadrivium. These consisted of grammar, rhetoric, logic; arithmetic, geometry with some astronomy, and the three philosophies, mental, moral, natural, of all of which Thomas Huxley, when making his inaugural address as the Lord Rector of Aberdeen University, said:

Thus their work, however imperfect and faulty judged by modern lights it may have been, brought them face to face with all the leading aspects of the many-sided mind of man. For these studies did really contain at any rate in embryo—sometimes it may be in caricature—what we now call philosophy, mathematical and physical science and art, and I doubt if the curriculum of any modern university shows so clear and generous a comprehension of what is meant by culture as the old trivium and quadrivium did.[6]

6 Thomas Huxley, Essay on "Universities: Actual and Ideal" in *Science and Education Essays*, (New York, D. Appleton & Co., 1896), p. 197.

After three years devoted to these studies, the student may, if he will, proceed to the study of medicine, provided always that during the prescribed time he devotes himself also to surgery which is a part of medicine. After this, but not before, he will be given a license to practice provided he has passed an examination in legal form as well as obtained a certificate from his teacher as to his studies. After having spent five years in study (we are just coming to the five-year requirement now) he shall not practice medicine until he has during a full year devoted himself to medical practice with the advice and under the direction of an experienced physician.

One would wonder just what would be the studies required but that also is nominated in the law:

In the medical schools the professors shall during these five years devote themselves to the recognized books, that is, the classical texts of Hippocrates as well as those of Galen, and shall teach not only theoretic but also practical medicine.

The law went further:

In every province of our kingdom which is under our legal authority we decree that two prudent and trustworthy men whose names must be sent to our court shall be appointed and bound by a formal oath, under whose inspection electuaries and syrups and other medicines be prepared according to law and only be sold after such inspection. In Salerno in particular we decree that this inspectorship shall be limited to those who have taken their degrees as master of physic.

In the universities of the Middle Ages, and especially those founded in western Europe in the twelfth and thirteenth centuries, this law of the Emperor Frederick II seems to have been taken as a model for the curriculum in school and the training apart from school in medicine. If we recall that as late as the seventies of the nineteenth century our medical schools in this country required but two terms of four months each for medical studies without any preliminary training being demanded, it will be easy to understand how much ahead of us were the medieval medical schools. Here in the United States you could come from the farm, or the mine, or before the mast, and if you could only read and write, and you didn't have to write any too well—the druggist would make out the prescription and perhaps do it better than the doctor—you would be admitted to the medical school and after eight months of study in two terms you were given a degree that was a license to practise medicine in any state in the Union.

President Eliot of Harvard has told the story in his *Harvard Memories* of how difficult a situation he found he was up against when he tried to make the medical school course consist of two terms of nine months each, with a written examination in nine subjects that had to be passed, though before that it had been considered that you need only pass five out of nine. The dean of the medical school said that the new, young president of the university would surely ruin the medical school because it could not be expected that the students should pass written examinations since a good many of them could not answer questions in writing in that way. Fortunately circumstances shaped themselves so that the overseers at Harvard stood sturdily behind the new, young president and Harvard maintained the primacy in medicine which it had been her privilege to maintain before that.

It is easy to understand that they were busy people during the Middle Ages to have been able to accomplish so much in every line of endeavor. They missed nothing in the development of the arts, and whatever they attempted they succeeded in very well, so that no wonder our age has gone back to the sincerest kind of admiration for them. The most interesting phase of this story of the thirteenth century is that the people of that time were so occupied with higher and better things that they had comparatively little time for war. I need scarcely say that we would like very much to find a formula of any kind that would keep this civilization of ours from being threatened by war to such a serious extent that we have begun to feel that culture is rushing headlong to destruction.

A commission was appointed at Harvard some time ago to study the number of wars that have occurred in various centuries in civilized countries in order, if possible, to get at the cause and the prevention of war. The report of the investigation made by that committee as it was given in the newspapers a few months ago, was that the greatest number of wars and the worst in their consequences had been fought in our own twentieth century, of which a while ago we were inclined to be so proud. The centuries nearest to us, to use the Miltonic phrase, achieved the "bad eminence" of having more wars than any other centuries. The eighteenth and nineteenth centuries were noteworthy in this regard. On the other hand, the century that had the least wars was the thirteenth, the very heart of the Middle Ages. The Harvard commission reported that in the thirteenth century there were six thousand more chances of dying in bed, or with your boots off, and there is a prejudice in favor of both of these circumstances as harmonizing with death, than in this twentieth century of ours.

Men of the thirteenth century were so occupied with mental and artistic achievement of various kinds, with preoccupation in art and the arts and crafts, with architecture and music, with literature and esthetic creation, with the making of things of beauty that are, as Keats declared, joys forever, with work in the precious metals and in wood and the base metals, with handsome textiles and marvelous paintings and sculpture, that they just did not have the time for the making of wars that we have at present. The lesson might well be worth-while. Our generation fails to occupy itself with the things of the mind and the heart and soul; hence the tendency for it to devote itself to things that are so much less worth-while.

V

THE SEARCH FOR LONGEVITY

BY

RAYMOND PEARL, Ph.D.

PROFESSOR OF BIOLOGY, THE JOHNS HOPKINS UNIVERSITY

V

THE SEARCH FOR LONGEVITY

I

THE available evidence indicates that during the last twenty-four hours something upwards of a sixth of a million fresh new human beings have appeared for the first time upon this earth as a whole. In other words, there has been delivered on our planet to-day well over 600 tons of that strange mixture of water, mineral salts and colloids called human, living substance. For delivery this material was neatly wrapped up in a lot of little packets that we call babies. These packets have been turned out to-day at a rate not much below two a second over the whole world. I speak of to-day's activities in the production department of human biology, merely because people like their statistics up to date. But the same sort of thing, in round figures, went on yesterday, and will occur again to-morrow, so we may as well focus attention on to-day's crop as any other.

Each one of these squalling blobs of protoplasm that starts to-day on the journey through time called the life span, will endeavor, with all its might and main, to make that journey last just as long as possible. For the will to live, the quest for longevity, is the most

deeply rooted and persistent of the biological characteristics of protoplasm organized into individuals. At the
beginning of each person's life this urge to survival, is
wholly unconscious, just a part of living, like digestion
or respiration; later on, this underlying protoplasmic
will to live, the vital momentum, will be supplemented
in the individual by a conscious search for longevity.
The great part of to-day's babies who manage to survive until they are somewhere in the twenties will
then begin to think a little about what they should
do to preserve their health so that they may keep on
living longer. Virtually all of them who live until
they are seventy years of age or upwards will think
about little else from that time on. For it is an odd
but profoundly true generalization of human biology
that the longer a human being has lived, the more
anxious and personally concerned he is, by and large,
to keep on living still longer. The octogenarian or
nonagenarian may be in wretched health and altogether having a bad time of it, but even so his normal
and sound instincts are for keeping on.

Incidentally, it is the almost universal lack of appetite for dying that makes the medical profession a
possible one. At the moment, as every one knows, the
profession is being wracked with discussions and torn
with dissensions over its economics. But if mankind
had not, from its remotest antiquity, been profoundly
of the opinion that the physician could be of significant help in the struggle to keep on living there
would be to-day no question of medical economics
to discuss. Physicians are employed, and sometimes

are paid, because people fear death and hope to keep on living. And doctors are not the only ones employed and paid for the same reasons. In spite of everything the honest, wise, and sincere members of the profession have been able to do, from the time when that arch quack Alexander of Abonutichus and his partner Cocconas practised their deplorable knavery down to the present, a horde of dubious charlatans of all complexions and degrees have fattened off humanity's distaste for dying. It has been revealed to many others besides the unworthy Alexander that, as Lucian said, "human life is under the absolute dominion of two mighty principles, fear and hope." Neither the art nor the science of medicine have as yet, alas, achieved an altogether complete understanding of life or of what to do to prolong it in the individual. The patient sometimes becomes impatient because this is so. Then, so compelling is his survival urge, he turns more often than would happen in a truly rational world to the ministrations of the quacks. Man's reason is evolutionally his most recent acquisition, so perhaps it is not altogether strange that it should be so easily overset by his baser biological instincts.

II

The duration of the journey through life that so many young hopefuls have started upon to-day will vary greatly among them. Some of the lot will end it to-morrow, so incomplete is their vital resource and so fragile their design for living. Others, a very few others, of the lot will be living a hundred years from now. The tired eyes of these will have seen many strange happenings in a dizzy world before their journey is done.

The pattern of these varying life journeys and the changes in that pattern in quite recent years are matters of considerable interest and are worth looking into on their own account as well as to give us a more solid ground for the further discussion of human longevity. The "order of dying" of a cohort of individuals all born at the same time is given with great accuracy by a device known as the life table, that combines mathematics and biology in a happy and useful mating. For purposes of the present discussion a certain function called the "survivorship" for two life tables has been put in a graphic form, on the supposition that the life journey, of which we have been speaking, consists in climbing a long and huge ladder. The first of the two life tables chosen for this treatment is one of the latest comprehensive American life tables. It combines into one single well-digested whole the mortality experience of the United States (exclusive of Texas and South Dakota) for the years 1929 to 1931, inclusive. This table was computed and published by Dublin and Lotka.[1] The sec-

---

[1] Louis I. Dublin and Alfred J. Lotka, *Length of Life. A Study of the Life Table* (New York, Ronald Press, 1926), pp. 14-17. The preliminary report of other official United States life tables for 1930, prepared in the Division of Statistical Research of the Bureau of the Census, was published in July, 1936, by Joseph A. Hill, *Vital Statistics—Special Reports*, I, pp. 389-399. For whites these tables are essentially similar to those given by Dublin and Lotka.

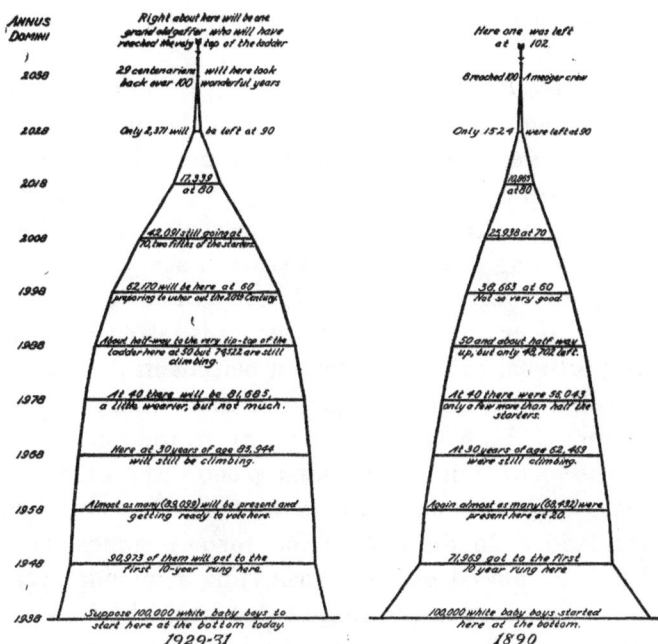

FIGURE 1.—The Ladder of Life, as it is shaped now (on the evidence of 1929-1931), and as it was in 1890, forty-eight years ago. For further explanation see text.

ond table to be depicted is that of Glover,[2] based upon the mortality experience of the State of Massachusetts in the year 1890. In both cases we shall deal with the order of dying of white males only. What is shown is the shape and dimensions of the ladders of life which the respective cohorts of white boy babies—

[2] James W. Glover, *United States Life Tables* 1890, 1901, 1910 and 1901-1910 (Washington, D. C., Government Printing Office, 1921), pp. 132-133.

that of 1930 and that of 1890—may be imagined as climbing.

The construction of the ladder is as follows: The total length (or height) of each ladder is the total *span* of life, which is about the same in each case— a little over 100 years. The rungs of the ladder are in each case set ten years of age apart, so that the bottom rung of each is at 10 years of age, the second rung at 20 years, and so on. The length of the rungs— or width or spread of the ladder—is, at each rung, proportional to the numbers of persons in the cohort who live long enough to get a foothold on that rung. Naturally, both ladders are drawn to the same scale in the picture. In both cases 100,000 just-born white male babies are supposed to start together climbing the ladder. In the case of the 1929-31 ladder there has been placed opposite each rung a calendar year date. This is meant to suggest that it will be a ladder of life much like the one here depicted that the white American boy babies born to-day will climb. This is not an entirely wild bit of prophecy, because past experience indicates that the ladder they will as- cend will almost certainly actually be as good as or bet- ter than this one, because it is not likely that medical and public health progress will stop abruptly. It is prog- ress in these two fields in the recent past that in large part has wrought the 1929-31 ladder of life into the shape seen in Figure 1. To be sure other things have been concerned in the matter too—such as improve- ments in the general conditions of living and of getting a living and in general education—but the forward strides of medical and public health knowledge and practice have surely been the most conspicuous causal elements involved.

It is at once evident that the two ladders, less than half a century apart in time, are quite different in shape. The one for 1930 has an air of broad substantiality, a solid structure that holds a lot of people. The 1890 one stands on the same base, but after the lowest rung is passed becomes a rather narrow, gangling thing, with much less of an air of solid stability; resembling strikingly the sort of ladder built for fruit picking, rather than the broad and heavy firemen's ladder on which human lives depend. At the 50-year rung the 1890 ladder of life accommodated fewer than half the persons who started the climb, while the 1930 ladder at the same point will hold almost three quarters of the starters.

III

In these pictures we see graphically how the prospects for the duration of the journey of life have been altered in the last fifty years or so, and for the better. The improvement has been great, and much credit is due to the medical and public health professions for the part they have played in bringing it about. But the pictures of the ladders do not make it entirely clear just how and wherein the improvement has been made. They give rather a broad general impression of the whole effect. In order to apprehend more clearly a very important, and often overlooked, point about this average improvement in the duration of the individual's life resort must be had to some other pictures, shown here as Figure 2.

These are pictures of life ladders, too, but of only their upper parts. Suppose we consider what happened subsequently to 10,000 white males who got to the 40-year rung of the 1890 ladder in comparison with 10,000 who will get to the same rung of the 1930 ladder; and then suppose we make the same comparison between 10,000 who got to the 70-year rung of the 1890 ladder and an equal number at the same position on the 1930 ladder.

It is at once evident from Figure 2 that the duration of the life journey after age 40 for those who have attained that age is, on the average, only slightly longer now than it was in 1890. According to the 1929-31 mortality experience 2.9 per cent of all those (males) reaching 40 lived to reach 90 years of age. But the 1890 experience shows that 2.7 per cent, or almost as many relatively, did the same then. The gain in the half century for the 40-year-old boys is wholly insignificant in any practical point of view.

Figure 2 further shows that those who attain the age of 70 now *actually do not do so well relatively,* on the average, in the way of further survival to still higher ages as did the stalwarts of 1890. At that time six hundred out of every 10,000 white males alive at age 70 lived on to 90 or more. Now, on the basis of the 1929-31 experience, only 563 manage this feat.

So it becomes plain that the important achievements in altering the shape of the ladder of life in the last 50 years, have been mainly in regard to the

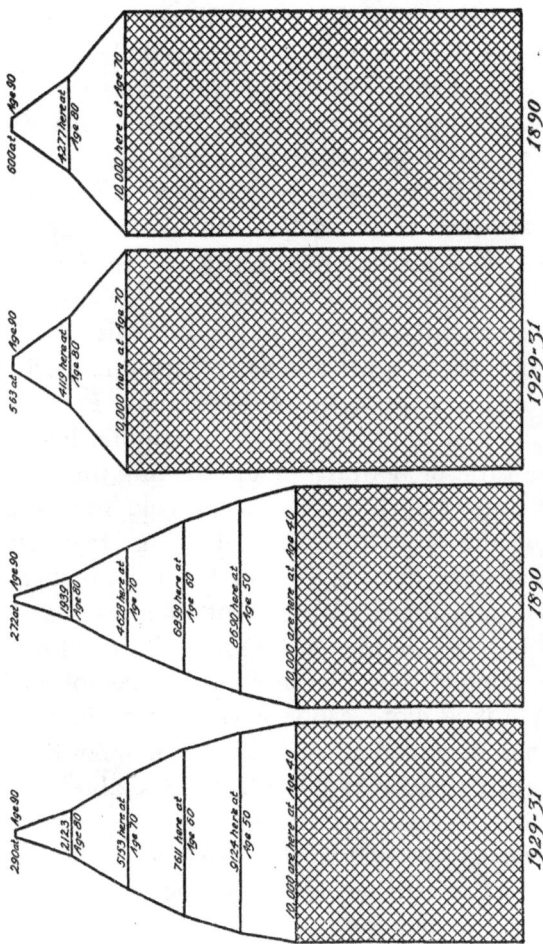

FIGURE 2.—The number of survivors at the later ages from an equal number starting at age 40 and at age 70, as shown by the U. S. life table (exclusive of Texas and South Dakota) of 1929-1931, and the Massachusetts life table of 1890. White Males.

lower rungs. And it is chiefly the lowest or 10-year rung that has been improved. In 1890 only 72 per cent of the boy babies starting got a foothold on that 10-year rung; now 91 per cent do. This is splendid and must certainly be warmly approved of by every small boy. But there is extremely little in it to bring cheer to the man at 40 who would like to buy an annuity and look forward to gloating over the issuing insurance company as a nonagenarian.

In the common way of thinking longevity really means living past 80 years, and great human longevity means being a nonagenarian or centenarian. Progress in medicine and improvement in the public health have done little or nothing about enabling the individual to achieve such a goal, as the cold statistical facts about the order of human dying make abundantly clear. The *span* of human life has *not* been lengthened, and there is no present prospect that it soon will be. The *average duration* of life is all that has been altered, and that has been accomplished chiefly by giving more babies a fairer start in life's journey than they used to have. Because more of them get by the early and very difficult hurdles, absolutely more of them survive at later ages. But the terms of the bet that any individual man aged 70 to-day can safely lay that he will be alive at 90 appear to be not quite as good as they were 50 years ago.

IV

What Everyman wants to know is whether there is not some sort of biological skullduggery that will, if he only knows what it is, enable him to make a surer and safer bet of this kind. There lies the real problem of the search for longevity. Why is it that some individuals alive at any given age will live thereafter longer than others? This is a biological question, and one of the most fundamental ones that science still has to worry over. In principle the duration of life of any individual is the net resultant of the interplay between his own innate biological make-up and the forces acting upon it, favorable or unfavorable, external and internal. This is a complete and sufficient logical statement of the case, but not so immediately useful as might be wished for the purpose of disappointing eager morticians. The practical searcher for individual longevity is not much interested in logical definitions. He is looking for more tangible help. What can be offered him?

One of the most often quoted things that Oliver Wendell Holmes ever said was that if one is setting out to achieve "three score years and twenty," the first thing to be done, "some years before birth, is to advertise for a couple of parents both belonging to long-lived families. Especially let the mother come of a race in which octogenarians and nonagenarians are very common phenomena." When this statement was made its only foundation was the general impression of a wise physician who spent his own life in a region where octogenarians and nonagenarians were common phenomena. Our practical searcher would like to know the extent or degree to which this impression has been supported by exact, quantitative investigation.

As the first and simplest approach to the question let us consider briefly the analysis of the pedigrees of persons who have actually achieved great longevity. For many years we have been collecting data about persons actually living at ages of 90 years and above. The collection now includes more than 2,000 such persons, for whom the personal and family records may be accepted as reliable and trustworthy, after having been thoroughly and critically checked. Many more cases than this have gone through our hands, but have been rejected for scientific study because they did not meet the standards of proof that were set up.

In 1934 my daughter and I [3] published a rather extensive and detailed analysis of 365 of these cases of proven extreme longevity. For each of these cases the ages at death of the six immediate ancestors (two parents and four grandparents) were known and recorded, as well as a great many other things about the person and the ancestors. As an example, the pedigree of one of these highly longevous persons is shown in Figure 3.

In this case the propositus (III, 4), living at the age of 100, was a Scottish seafaring man, who married and "settled down" at the age of 39. His immediate ancestry is very remarkable in point of longevity. His father (II, 1) and his maternal grandmother (I, 2) died as the result of accidents. His two children

[3] Raymond Pearl and Ruth D. Pearl, *The Ancestry of the Long-Lived* (Baltimore, Johns Hopkins, 1934).

(IV, 1 and IV, 3) who died at early ages, met their end by drowning.

At the top of the chart the mysterious word TIAL is

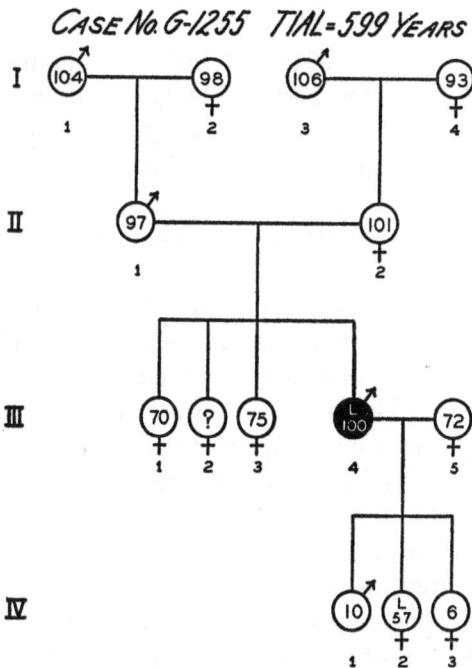

FIGURE 3.—Pedigree of a centenarian. In this pedigree the person under discussion (the propositus) is indicated by a solid sex sign. Figures within the circles of the sex signs indicate the ages at death in years, except where there is an L above the age figure, which means that the person was living at the time of record, and at the indicated age in years.

merely an abbreviation for "total immediate ancestral longevity," and is used to designate the sum of the ages at death of the parents and grandparents.

Thus in the present case $104 + 98 + 106 + 93 + 97 + 101 = 599$ years. It is safe to say that few human beings have ever had an authentic TIAL number higher than this.

But how much lower are the TIALs of ordinary people, just "run-of-mine" folk who do not themselves live, on the average, longer than the average of the general population? To get an approximate answer to this question, and to have a group to compare with the highly longevous group of nonagenarians and centenarians we assembled, entirely at random so far as concerned their own ages, a group of 136 living persons all six of whose immediate ancestors (parents and grandparents) were dead at the time of observation, and for each of whom the age at death was known and recorded. This seems as fair a group for comparing TIALs with the longevous group as it is humanly possible to get. This comparison group had an average living age of 48.75 years, and contained 29 persons over 60 at the time of observation, 6 over 70, and 1 over 80. The average age of the group was almost 16 years higher than that of the living white population of the United States in 1930.

How does the ancestral longevity of this group of ordinary folk compare with that of the élite group of extraordinary long-livers, the nonagenarians and centenarians? Figure 4 gives the answer in graphic form.

From this diagram it is seen that, on the average, each single immediate ancestor, father, mother, grand-

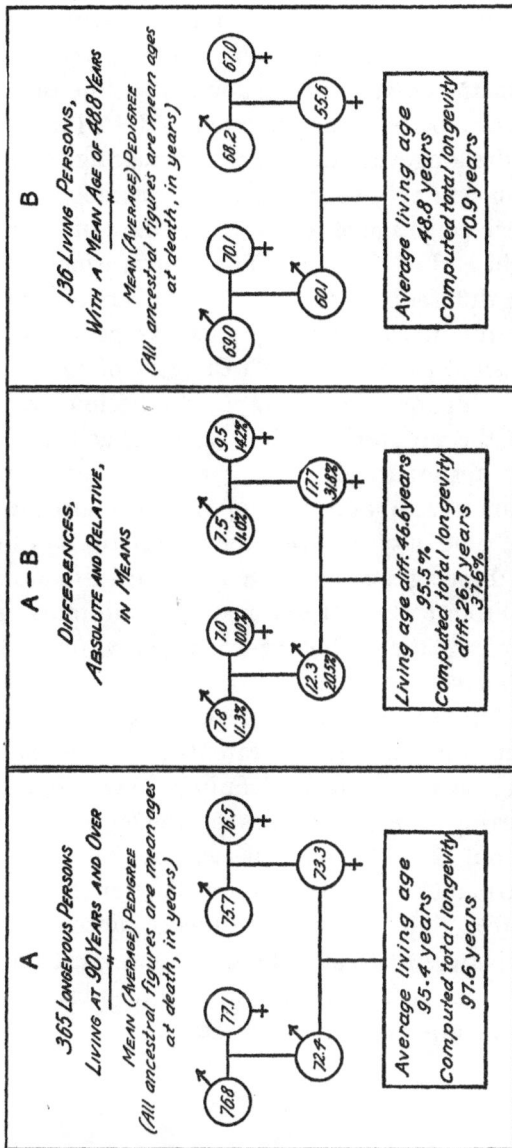

FIGURE 4.—Influence of immediate ancestors upon mean (average) longevity.

father, or grandmother, of the extremely longevous persons of panel A on the left side, was longer-lived than the corresponding ancestor of the ordinary persons of panel B on the right side. Thus the fathers of the longevous died at the average age of 72.4 years. This was 12.3 years older, or over 20 per cent, than the average age of the fathers of the panel B folk at the right end of the chart. The central panel, A—B, gives the differences, in absolute numbers of years (upper figures in each sex sign) and as percentages of the panel B means, for each category of the six immediate ancestors. The "computed total longevity" figures for the propositi in the rectangles at the bottom are the resultants of adding to the mean number of years the A and B propositi had already lived at the time of observation the expectations of life proper to those ages, as given in a standard life table.

From this chart two results indubitably emerge regarding the influence of heredity upon longevity, namely:

(*a*) People who achieve extreme longevity have immediate ancestors (parents and grandparents) who are, on the average, definitely longer lived than the corresponding ancestors of the general run of the population. This is true without exception for each particular category of immediate ancestors.

(*b*) This hereditary influence promoting longevity is between two and three times as great relatively for parents as it is for grandparents, so far as the results of this investigation indicate.

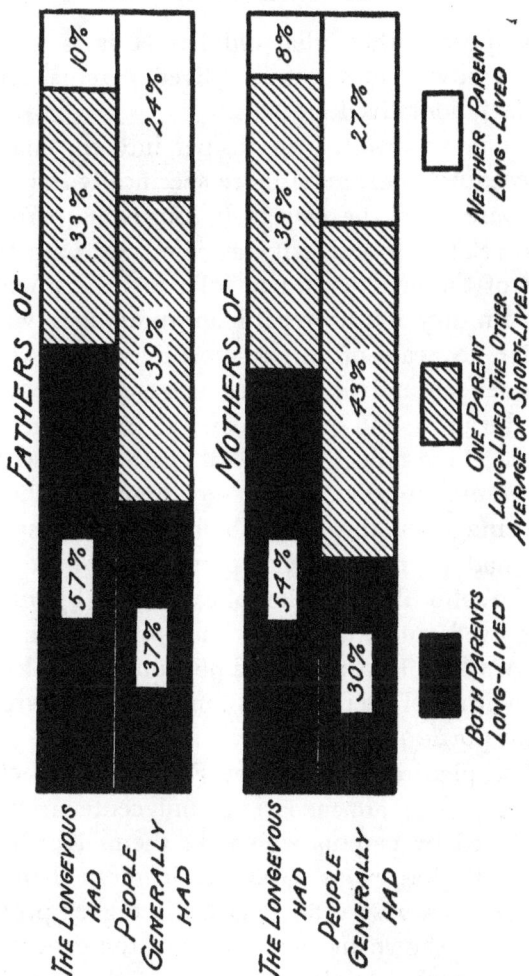

FIGURE 5.—How the Parents of the Long-Lived are Bred: The percentage distribution, relative to the nature of the parental matings producing them, of the fathers and of the mothers of (a) an extremely longevous group (nonagenarians and centenarians), and (b) a defined sample of people generally.

It appears, then, that old Dr. Holmes was sound in his advice to select long-lived parents, and particularly long-lived mothers.

Let us now go a little deeper into the matter, by proceeding to examine more specifically how each of the *parents* of the extremely longevous persons was bred relative to longevity, as compared with the parents of the general run of folk. For the purposes of this inquiry let us regard an individual who dies under 50 years of age as short-lived; one who dies between 50 and 69 years as average or mediocre in life duration, and one who dies at 70 or over as long-lived. These ranges in general agree fairly with common-sense opinion and usage. Figure 5 shows the percentages of the fathers and mothers respectively that had (a) both of *their* parents long-lived (shown by the solid black portion of each bar; (b) one parent long-lived and the other mediocre or short-lived (shown by the cross-hatched portion of each bar); and (c) neither of their parents long-lived (shown by the white portion of each bar).

The picture presented by Figure 5 is precise and striking. The nonagenarians and centenarians were produced by parents who were themselves bred out of wholly longevous parentage in more than half of all the cases observed—a markedly higher proportion than that shown by the parents of the general population sample. At the other end of the genetic scale the opposite is true. Fewer than half as many proportionally of the nonagenarians and centenarians as of persons generally were produced by parents who themselves had no longevous parentage whatever. It seems clear beyond question or doubt that breeding counted mightily in the production of these nonagenarians and centenarians.

Let us now turn to another method of approach, and a wholly different material, to get still another view of the importance of inheritance in the quest for longevity. Suppose one were to go out and collect entirely at random every single case possible to find of children dying before they were five years old— extremely short-lived human beings in fact, who were unable to get far in the pleasant business of living either because they were inherently bad biological eggs literally or figuratively, or because they never had a fair chance to live on account of a bad environment associated with parental poverty or ignorance or vice. Now suppose further that we followed the fathers of these poor creatures along through their whole lives and set down in the record their ages at death when they (the fathers) finally died. It would then be possible to construct a life table for the category of *fathers of persons dying under 5 years of age*. Having done all this, suppose we next did precisely the same thing for a group of fathers of persons who did not die until they were 80 years old or more —in other words, a group of old gaffers with demonstrated great powers of living, which powers may conceivably have arisen from their innately superior biological make-up, or from great good luck combined with good sense in their choice of victuals and drink, or from always wearing their rubbers when it rained and woolies when it was cold, and so on through the entire list of precepts and superstitions thought to promote longevity. When the data had been collected and the computations made we should then be in possession of a life table for the category of *fathers of persons dying at 80 and over years of age.*[4]

How will these two life tables compare with each other? Figure 6 shows the answer so far as concerns the expectation of life (or average-after-lifetime) at four selected ages: 20, 40, 60, and 80 years.

It is at once evident that, so far as concerns the present material involving well over a hundred thousand life years' exposure to risk, the long-lived children had fathers who were much longer-lived than the fathers of short-lived children. The figures at the tops of the bars give the expectations of life at the ages indicated at the bottoms of the bars. Thus the average *total* duration of life from birth of the fathers of children dying at ages of 80 and over was $58.5 + 20 = 78.5$ years.

Corresponding life tables for mothers tell the same sort of story, as is shown in Figure 7.

The *relative* excess in life duration of the parents of long-lived as compared with short-lived children is very considerable. Thus the mean-after-lifetime of *fathers* of children dying (or living) at ages of 80

<hr>

[4] For details regarding the construction of these and the life tables to be discussed below see R. Pearl, "Studies on Human Longevity. IV. The Inheritance of Longevity." *Human Biology*, III, 1931, 245-269.

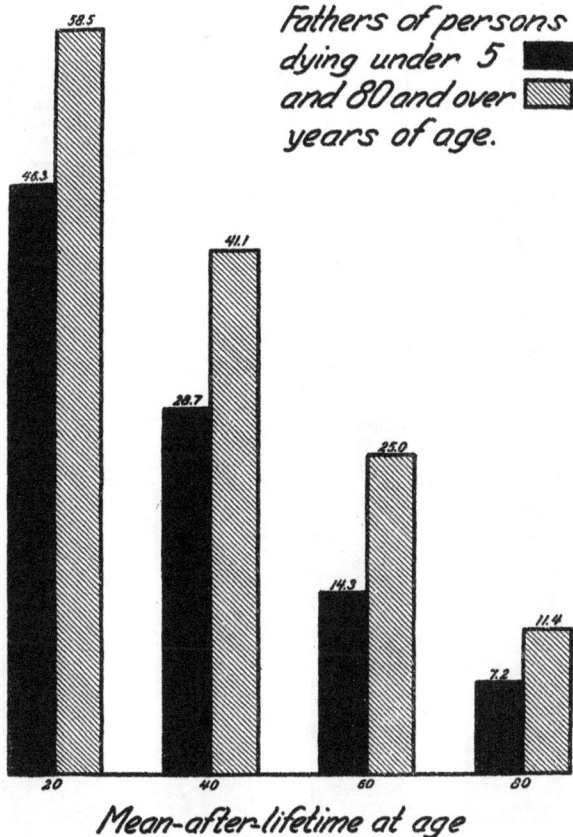

FIGURE 6.—Expectation of life in years (mean-after-lifetime) at ages 20, 40, 60, and 80, of fathers of children dying (a) under 5 years of age (solid bars) and (b) 80 and over years of age (cross-hatched bars).

and over is about 26 per cent greater at age 20; 43 per cent greater at age 40; 75 per cent greater at age 60; and 58 per cent greater at age 80, than the mean-

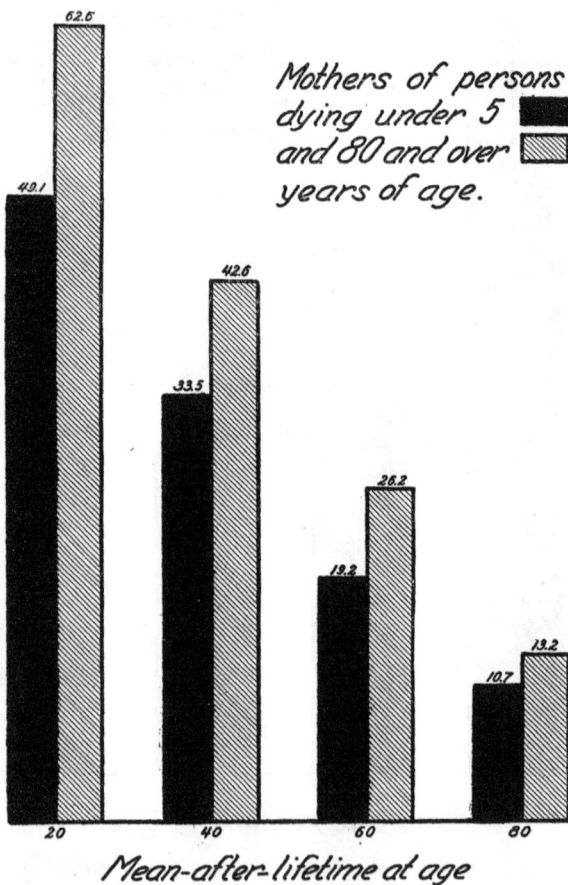

FIGURE 7.—Like Figure 6, but for mothers.

after-lifetime at the same ages of fathers of children dying under 5. The corresponding excesses in expectation of life of mothers are 27 per cent at age 20; 27 per cent at age 40; 36 per cent at age 60; and 23 per cent at age 80. The suggestion plainly is that right away through the whole life span the parents of very long-lived children appear to be persons of superior biological constitution, as evidenced by their ability to keep on living.

What now of the situation turned the other way about? How will the respective life tables compare if we construct them for the *children* of short-lived, moderately long-lived and very long-lived parents? This we have done for *sons* as a class, with the results shown in Figure 8.

Plainly the results of these life tables for sons confirm the conclusions derived from those for fathers and mothers that have just been examined. As we pass upwards through the three broad classes of paternal longevity the expectation of life of the sons at all ages steadily rises. The expectation of life of the sons of short-lived fathers is less than that of the sons of moderately longevous fathers, and still less than that of the sons of extremely long-lived fathers. Thus at age 60 the sons of very long-lived fathers (80 and over) have a further average expectation of life nearly 40 per cent greater than that of sons whose fathers died before age 50.

It seems unnecessary to present further evidence to demonstrate the great significance of genetic factors in determining individual differences in the length of human life. The inherited biological constitution of each individual human being—his or her genetically determined inherent viability—is beyond question one of the major determiners of the probable length of that person's life. It is not, however, the sole or absolute determiner. Obviously any one can behave in such a way that his or her genetic birthright in longevity is prevented from coming to its full expression. Prematurely taking one's own life is perhaps the most nearly perfect example. On the other hand, the general effect of public health and sanitary measures is to create and promote such conditions of living as will permit the greatest possible number of people to bring as nearly as possible to complete realization and expression the inherent viability with which they have been genetically endowed. In the changing shapes of the ladder of life shown earlier, it has been seen how great the progress has been in this respect for the earlier years, and how little for the later years of the life span. This suggests, in the light of the evidence regarding the inheritance factors in longevity, two conclusions that may be of considerable significance. The first is that there exist broad classes of human beings differentiated from each other in their innate endowments in respect of inherent viability, one class being short and the other being long of this important quality. The second suggested conclusion is that improving the environmental circumstances of living can do, and has done, a great deal more for the first class than for the second in the way of increased longevity. It appears probable that there is now, and always has been in past ages, a class of human beings by nature so abundantly endowed in the matter of viability that they have always, as a statistical group, so nearly realized their

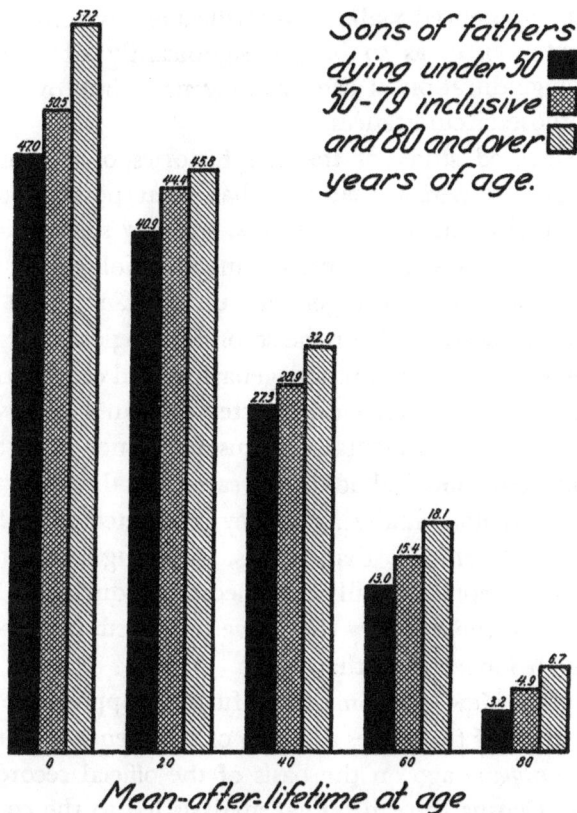

FIGURE 8.—Expectation of life in years (mean-after-lifetime) at ages 0 (birth), 20, 40, 60, and 80 years, of the *sons* of fathers dying (a) under 50 years of age (solid bars); (b) between 50 and 79 years of age (double cross-hatched bars); and (c) 80 and over years of age (single cross-hatched bars).

innate potential viability regardless of environmental circumstances as to be not significantly affected in average duration of life by any general improvement of those circumstances.

Detailed study of the life histories of extremely longevous persons, such as has been possible with our collection of such records, strongly suggests that nonagenarians and centenarians are biologically differentiated from the general run of mankind in the manner postulated for the second biological class just described. As a group nonagenarians and centenarians have definitely *not* led protected lives in specially favorable environmental circumstances; nor have they had better medical advice or care than the generality of men; nor, finally have they conducted their lives more hygienically than others, according to the rules and precepts generally regarded as conducive to long life. On the contrary they have just lived, but lived a much longer time than most.

This view of the matter is further supported by an analysis of the causes of death of nonagenarians, made some years ago on the basis of the official records of the Census Bureau.[5] That analysis led to the conclusion that nonagenarians are a selected lot of people. They are the ultimate survivors after all the rest of mankind has gone, unable to meet the vicissitudes of life and keep on living. Nonagenarians come to be

[5] Raymond Pearl and T. Raenkham, "Studies on Human Longevity. V. Constitutional Factors in Mortality at Advanced Ages." *Human Biology*, IV, 1932, 80-118.

such because they have organically superior consti-
tutions, resistent to infections, soundly organized to
function efficiently as a whole organism and keep on
doing it for a very long time. Observations on mortality at ages indicate that throughout life infections
and other harmful environmental forces are, on the
whole, tending to take off the weaker and leave the
stronger. Medical knowledge and skill, improved
sanitation and better conditions of life generally have
been and are, able to prevent an increasingly larger
amount of what may be called premature mortality
before age 50, let us say. Especially have these agencies
been able to reduce the lethal effects of infection,
or at least to postpone to a later part of the life span
their fatal action. But ultimately there is left a group
of extremely old people, for whom on the whole
infections have no particular terrors. In all the early
part of their lives they have been able successfully
to resist infections, and to a remarkable degree still
are in extreme old age. These people eventually die,
to be sure. But a great part of them die, not because
the noxious forces of the environment kill them, but
because their vital machinery literally breaks down,
and particularly that important part of it—the circulatory system.

v

Evidence has been presented indicating that genetic
factors are important in determining individual
longevity. It has further been suggested that these
genetic influences manifest themselves in relation to

longevity primarily through the general biological constitution of the individual, so far as can be judged on the basis of present knowledge regarding this complex and difficult problem.

There will now be presented for the first time, in necessarily condensed form, some results of an investigation now in progress that appear to throw additional light on the problem of constitution in relation to longevity. The problem attacked may be put in this way: Suppose that one were able to make fairly thorough and complete studies, medical, anthropometric and genetic, of adult persons in a state of health at the time of observation, then follow them individually till they died, and then finally determine and record the causes of their deaths individually. Would it then be possible to isolate and differentiate any characteristic exhibited at the time of original observation years before, from which could have been predicted *then* who were destined to be the long-lived and who the short-lived, had the original observer been as wise before the event as afterwards? In other words, is it possible by any sort of examination or study of healthy adult individuals to predict which ones are destined for a long subsequent life and which will exhibit no marked powers of further survival?

At the expense of considerable time and labor records have been collected upon this question, and some of them have been analyzed. In particular we have studied rather thoroughly 386 white males from this point of view. These individuals were originally observed and recorded at ages ranging from 20 to over 60 years; 193 of them proved in the event to be long-lived, in the sense that each one of them outlived in greater or smaller degree the expectation of life (mean-after-lifetime) for his age when observed, according to Dublin and Lotka's 1929-31 life tables referred to above. All white males in our records fulfilling this condition of survivorship greater than that expected from the life table were taken for study without any selection. Then as a partner for each one of these 193 long-lived males there was taken from the record a white male of the same decade of age, who died *before* reaching the expected degree of survivorship proper to his age as set forth in the Dublin and Lotka life tables. All these 386 persons died in the end of some form of cardiovascular disease —that is of heart disease in one or another of its forms or of some affection of the arteries or veins.

So then in sum, what we have are two groups of white males of the same age distribution and in a state of health at the time of observation, all of whom died of diseases characterized by structural or functional breakdown or inadequacy of the circulatory system. One of these groups was definitely longer-lived than the average of American men at the present time, while the other group was definitely shorter-lived than the average. In what respects, if any, did the two groups differ from one another before either displayed any discernible evidence of cardiovascular disease? Table I and Figure 9 give the more important aspects of the answer to this question.

TABLE I

CONSTITUTIONAL DIFFERENCES BETWEEN LONG-LIVED AND SHORT-LIVED WHITE MALES WHEN OBSERVED IN A STATE OF HEALTH PRIOR TO THE ONSET OF THE CARDIOVASCULAR DISEASES THAT EVENTUALLY LED TO DEATH

PART A. *Age and Physiological Characteristics*

Cause of death, group and differences	Mean (average) value of characteristic					
	Age at observation (yrs.)	Age at death (yrs.)	Actual survival (yrs.)	Percentage of expected survival (yrs.)	Pulse rate (per minute)	Systolic blood pressure
Long-lived ($N = 193$)	40.09	76.59	36.49	123.45	73.45	133.89
Short-lived ($N = 193$)	39.56	50.27	10.69	35.45	74.62	131.22
Difference	+0.53±.71	+26.32±.50	+25.80±.63	—	−1.17±.29	+2.67±1.74
Difference as per cent of short-lived mean	+1.34	+52.36	+241.35	—	−1.57	+2.03

Part B. *Somatological Characteristics*

Cause of death, group and differences	Mean (average) value of characteristic						
	Stature (cm.)	Body weight (kg.)	Body weight ratio (kg.)	Chest girth at expiration (cm.)	Chest expansion (cm.)	Umbilical girth (cm.)	Habitus index (cm.)
Long-lived (N = 193)	173.80	70.27	4.04	86.62	9.06	85.05	98.77
Short-lived (N = 193)	174.09	74.56	4.28	89.61	9.55	86.47	101.09
Difference	−0.29 ± .43	−4.29 ± .68	−0.24	−2.89 ± .48	−0.47 ± .21	−1.42 ± .62	−2.32
Difference as per cent of short-lived mean	−0.17	−5.75	−5.60	−3.23	−5.13	−1.64	——

Part C. *Genetic Data*

Cause of death, group and differences	Mean (average) value of characteristic					
	Percentage of parents living at time of observation	Percentage of sibship living at time of observation	Percentage of total sibship dying in infancy	Percentage of all parents and sibs dead of cardiovascular diseases	Percentage of all parents and sibs dead of respiratory diseases	Percentage of all parents and sibs dead of diseases of alimentary tract
Long-lived (N = 193)	48.96	73.71	9.15	3.00	5.33	3.43
Short-lived (N = 193)	41.58	80.56	5.72	4.92	4.37	2.98
Difference	+7.38	−6.84	+3.43	−1.92	+0.96	+0.45

Considering Part A of the table, it is seen that while the two groups were substantially *identical* in average age at observation (approximately 40 years) the long-lived group lived thereafter more than 26 years or over 52 per cent *longer* than did the short-lived group. The actual survival of the first group was 123 per cent of life table expectation, while that of the second group was only about 35 per cent of life table expectation.

At the time of observation the average pulse rate per minute was, by an absolutely small but statistically significant amount *slower* in those destined for long life than in those who were to live less than a third as long a time. Furthermore the long-lived group exhibited at observation an average systolic blood pressure slightly over 2 per cent *higher* than did the short-lived group, a difference that is, however, statistically insignificant. The average blood pressure in both groups, it will be noted, was well within what is regarded as the clinically normal range for persons of an average age of about 40 years. But the number in the long-lived group for which blood pressure readings were available was very small (27 cases only), so that altogether the findings relative to blood pressure depend upon only 54 individuals in total. A satisfactory appraisal of the situation relative to blood pressure differences between long-lived and short-lived groups will have to wait on the slow accumulation of additional data.

In physical characteristics of the body (Part B) the two groups were of substantially *identical* average stature, but the long-lived group *weighed,* on the average, nearly 6 per cent *less* than the short-lived group, again a statistically significant difference. Furthermore the long-lived averaged to be *smaller* in chest girth (at expiration) and in girth at the level of the navel (umbilical girth) than the short-lived. Also, as shown by the habitus index,[6] the long-lived group on the average was *less* of the pyknic type in body build than the short-lived group—in other words the long-livers tended to be more like Don Quixote and the short-livers more like Sancho Panza in their bodily structure.

The long-lived group had over 7 per cent *more,* on the average, of their parents alive at the time of observation than did the short-lived group, indicating a sounder inheritance in respect of longevity. On the other hand, *fewer* of the brothers and sisters of the long-lived, on the average, were still living when the observations were made, than was the case with the short-lived. This suggests that natural selection had operated more stringently in the sibships containing the long-lived persons, an interpretation that is supported by the higher infant mortality rate that had manifested itself in the sibships of the long-lived.

[6] $\text{Habitus index} = \dfrac{100 \ (\text{Chest girth at expiration} + \text{umbilical girth})}{\text{Stature}}$

This somatological index, which appears not to have been used hitherto, is proving to be a very useful one in classifying variation in bodily habitus (Kretschmerian typology). The asthenic type of body build leads to a relatively low index, and the pyknic type to a relatively high one. It is intended to publish soon in another place a detailed discussion of this index.

Finally, and more specifically from the genetic side, the long-lived group had *fewer* proportionately of their parents and sibs dead of cardiovascular diseases at the time of observation than did the short-lived.

Figure 9 sums up graphically some of the results of this constitutional study.

In general it appears, so far as may be judged from the present sample, that there is a definite possibility that long-lived persons as a group can be statistically differentiated from short-lived persons in respect of a number of structural, physiological, and genetic characteristics, long before they are going to die and while they are still in sound health. It would be unwise to generalize much further than this at present. More work needs to be done, and we propose to continue doing it just as rapidly and extensively as can be managed. It is a laborious and expensive sort of research, and the resources available to us for its support are so meager that progress is distressingly slow. But the results already achieved seem clearly to indicate that we have opened up here a line of approach to the problems of human longevity that gives promise of eventually yielding results of considerable significance, both theoretical and practical. We have made similar analyses to the one here presented for two smaller groups of long-lived and short-lived persons dying respectively of cancer and of pneumonia, with extremely suggestive results; but the cases available are still too small to warrant even preliminary publication at present.

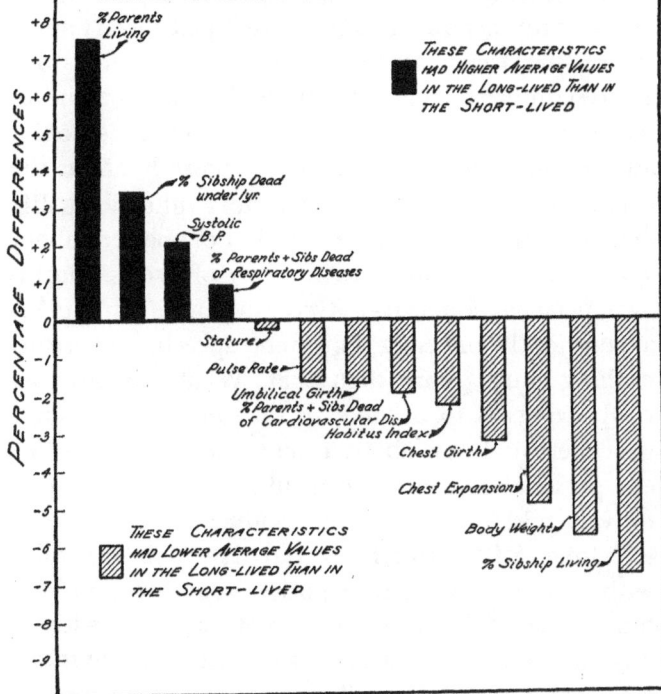

FIGURE 9.—Some relative differences in constitution between long-lived and short-lived white males. For further description see text.

VI

Up to this point the discussion has been almost entirely of the innate, constitutional elements concerned in the determination of individual life duration. It is now time that some attention be devoted to the environmental aspects of the picture. Here is where the eager searcher for longevity finds his greatest interest. For while he will admit that in an academic or philosophical point of view it is doubtless desirable to know as much as possible about the hereditary and constitutional factors influencing life duration, still these are after all not matters about which he can do much in the way of promoting his own personal longevity. "Choosing one's parents" is a sufficiently amusing figure of speech, but really nothing much more than that. What our searcher really wants is to be able to do something effective right here and now about a matter of such transcendent personal concern. He would like to be authoritatively told how he should conduct his life so as to live long. Still better he would like to be provided with some pleasant pill or potion guaranteed to keep him going until he reaches ninety at least, without any bother about what he eats or drinks in the meantime, or whether he bundles up well when he goes out in the cold. Best of all he would like to be supplied with some of the authentic juice that flows from the Fountain of Perpetual Youth. Since mankind started making literary records of his thoughts and aspirations the search for that elusive spring has been earnestly prosecuted. Many people have figured out just what it would look like when it was found. One of the most charming and delightful of its many portrayals serves as the frontispiece of a rather rare book that is one of the gems of an extensive collection of tracts and treatises dealing with longevity down through the ages. The title page and frontispiece of this book are shown in facsimile in Figures 10 and 11.

One notes the triumphant and smug satisfaction with which his conductor is telling the weary and skeptical old physician in the lower left foreground, who may be Æsculapius himself: "There, you doubting old fuddy-duddy, I said it was here, and *here it is!* See for yourself!" In the right foreground is evident the almost obscene eagerness of the old boys just arrived to guzzle the precious fluid gushing from the fountain, while the bloated Saurian leers up at them and gets his share. In the distant background we get a glimpse of the garden in which so much of humanity as was there remained perpetually youthful, until the lady unfortunately committed a technical error. The fauna of the environs of the fountain is characteristically reptilian. Of the four Orders of the Class Reptilia three are represented—the *Loricata* (Crocodiles and Alligators), the *Chelonia* (Tortoises and Turtles), and the *Squamata* (Lizards and Snakes). The only Order omitted is the *Rhyncocephalia,* which contains only one form, the famous *Tuatera* found in the islands of Cook Strait, New Zealand. This seems an excusable omission, because New Zealand has always been so far away from the center of

HISTOIRE
DES PERSONNES
QUI ONT VECU
PLUSIEURS SIECLES,
ET QUI ONT RAJEUNI:
AVEC LE SECRET
DU RAJEUNISSEMENT.

Tiré d'Arnauld de Villeneuve.

Et des Régles pour se conserver en santé,
& pour parvenir à un grand âge

Par Mr. DE LONGEVILLE HARCOUET.

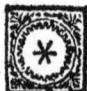

A PARIS,
Chez la Veuve CARPENTIER, & LAU-
RENT LE COMTE. 1716.

AVEC APPROBATION ET PRIVILEGE.

Se vend A BRUXELLES,
Chez JEAN LEONARD, Libraire &
Imprimeur rue de la Cour.

FIGURE 10.—Facsimile of the title page of Harcouet's *Histoire.*

things. It will also be noted that an elephant is emerging from the trees in the background. This is to round out the lesson of the picture as a whole; because, of all mammals except man, the elephant is the longest lived. The reptilia, of course, have always been noted for longevity. The banner borne by the two rocs at the top of the picture is an anachronism, plainly put in as a sop to conservative respectability. For if we really had access to the Fountain of Perpetual Youth who would worry about health?

Unfortunately we cannot serve a draft from the Fountain of Youth on this occasion. Lacking this the best that can be done is to discuss some of the environmental factors that have been thought to be, or in fact are, importantly concerned in the achievement of longevity. Only those will be chosen for discussion about which there exists definite scientific evidence, pertinent to the point at issue.

Of all such factors the use of alcoholic beverages has probably been most discussed. The problem of the effect of such usage upon longevity has excited violent and unreasoning prejudice on the part of large numbers of people. They contend that alcohol always and everywhere shortens the lives of its users. There is much evidence, experimental, statistical, and actuarial, that this is not a universally valid generalization. This evidence does not make the slightest impression upon those who believe, that is to say *have faith*, that the generalization is valid. So an impasse results. So far as I am aware there has been constructed only once a set of life tables for classes

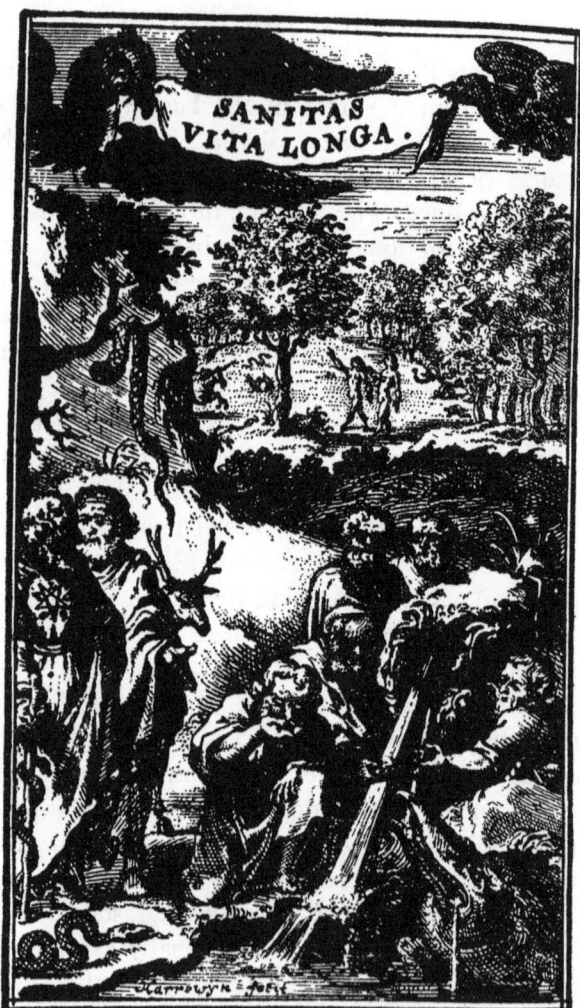

FIGURE 11.—Facsimile of the frontispiece of Harcouet's *Histoire*, depicting the Fountain of Youth. Original size of engraved area 110 x 66 mm.

of persons homogeneous in respect of their habits relative to alcoholic indulgence, and based upon critically adequate and pertinent data collected at first hand.[7] Those life tables lead to the general conclusion graphically depicted in Figure 12.

That conclusion is that moderate drinking does not significantly shorten life when compared with total abstention from alcohol, while heavy drinking does seriously diminish the length of life.

These results have been accepted by some, and rejected by other equally sincere, equally honest, and intelligent groups of people, who however differ widely in their emotions and sentiments regarding the use of alcohol by man as a beverage. Nothing further can be done about the case. Presumably every one is already a component of one or the other of these two groups.

Let us turn next to the use of tobacco and longevity. This usage is probably, along with that of alcohol, one of the most wide-spread amongst humanity relative to substances or materials that are not, in themselves, necessary to the maintenance of life as is food. Is the smoking of tobacco associated statistically with any impairment of the normal expectation of life, or with an improvement of it, or is there no measurable association one way or the other? This question, too, has excited controversy, though not so violent as that over alcohol. It is the intention to present now for the first time a small part of the hitherto unpub-

[7] Raymond Pearl, *Alcohol and Longevity* (New York, Alfred A. Knopf, 1926).

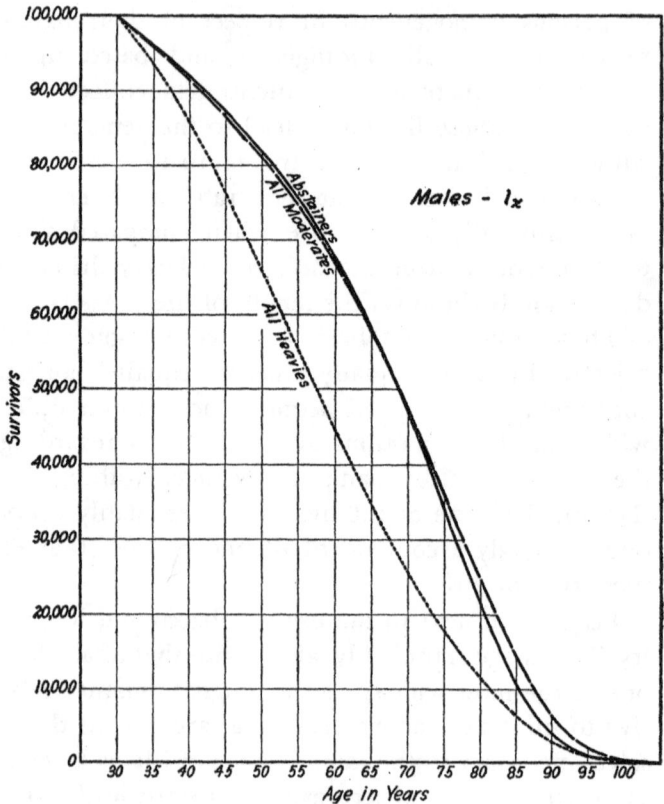

FIGURE 12.—The number of surviving males out of 100,000 starting together at age 30, in three drinking categories: (a) abstainers (solid line), (b) moderate drinkers (dash line), and (c) heavy drinkers (dot line).

lished results of an investigation of this problem.[8] This investigation, like the preceding one on alcohol, has been carried out with painstaking care, and such critical acumen, judgment, and fairness, as my collaborators and I possess. The data were collected at first hand *ad hoc*. Their accuracy as to the relative degree of habitual usage of tobacco, and as to the ages of the living at risk, and of the dead at death can be guaranteed. The figures to be presented deal only with white males, and with the usage of tobacco by smoking. The material falls into three categories, as follows: *non-users* of tobacco, of whom there were 2,094; *moderate smokers,* of whom there were 2,814; and *heavy smokers,* of whom there were 1,905. In other words, the results presented here are based upon the observation of 6,813 men in total. These are not large numbers from an actuarial point of view, but are sufficient to be probably indicative of the trends that would be shown by more ample material. Naturally the men included in the observation were an unselected lot except as to their tobacco habits. That is to say they were taken at random, and then all sorted into categories relative to tobacco usage. For each of the three categories of tobacco usage, complete life tables from age 30 on to the end of the life span have been constructed.

It is intended to publish eventually in detail the results of this investigation. Here there can be presented only a condensed table, which gives the survivorship (l_x) values, at 5-year intervals from age 30 on, for the three usage categories.

8 Since this lecture was delivered there has been published a further account of these life tables (Raymond Pearl, "Tobacco and Longevity," *Science,* LXXXVII, 1938, 216-217.)

TABLE II

THE NUMBER OF SURVIVORS, AT 5-YEAR AGE INTERVALS STARTING AT AGE 30, OF (A) 100,000 WHITE MALES WHO WERE NON-USERS OF TOBACCO; (B) 100,000 WHO WERE MODERATE SMOKERS BUT DID NOT CHEW TOBACCO OR TAKE SNUFF; AND (C) 100,000 WHO WERE HEAVY SMOKERS BUT DID NOT CHEW OR

TAKE SNUFF

AGE	NUMBER OF SURVIVORS		
	Non-users	Moderate	Heavy
30	100,000	100,000	100,000
35	95,883	95,804	90,943
40	91,546	90,883	81,191
45	86,730	85,129	71,665
50	81,160	78,436	62,699
55	74,538	70,712	54,277
60	66,564	61,911	46,226
65	57,018	52,082	38,328
70	45,919	41,431	30,393
75	33,767	30,455	22,338
80	21,737	19,945	14,494
85	11,597	10,987	7,865
90	4,573	4,686	3,292
95	1,320	1,366	938

The figures of Table II are shown graphically in Figure 13.

The net result is obvious. In this group of nearly 7,000 men the smoking of tobacco was associated definitely with an impairment of life duration, and the amount or degree of this impairment increased as the habitual amount of smoking increased. The contrast between the life tables relative to the implied effects upon longevity of moderate smoking, on the

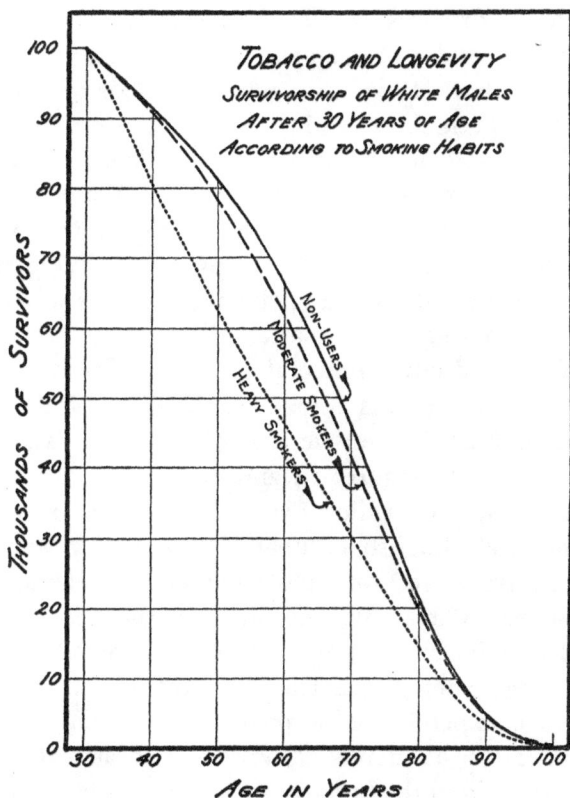

FIGURE 13.—The survivorship lines of life tables for white males falling into three categories relative to the usage of tobacco. (a) non-users (solid line); (b) moderate smokers (dash line), (c) heavy smokers (dot line).

one hand, and the moderate use of alcoholic beverages, on the other hand, is very striking. The moderate smokers in this material are definitely shorter lived than the total abstainers from tobacco; the

moderate drinkers are not significantly worse or better off in respect of longevity than the total abstainers
from alcohol. Heavy indulgence in either tobacco or
alcohol is associated with a very poor life table, but
the life table for heavy smokers is definitely worse
than that for heavy drinkers up to about age 60.
Thereafter to the end of the life span the heavy
smokers do a relatively better job of surviving than
the heavy drinkers. But neither group has anything
to boast about in the matter of longevity.

The third environmental problem to be discussed
may be put in this way: Does hard physical labor
shorten life? The answer to this question is shown
graphically in Figures 14 and 15.

The data [9] on which Figures 14 and 15 are based
come from English occupational mortality statistics
which are as accurate and comprehensive as any in
existence. The results indicate that there is a direct
and definite relation between the magnitude of the
age specific death rates from age 40 to 45 on, and the
average expenditure of physical energy in occupation, *after* accidental deaths and deaths directly
resulting from the hazards of each of the several occupations have been deducted. This relation is of the
sort that associates high mortality with hard physical
labor. The relationship prevails whether the labor is
performed chiefly indoors or chiefly outdoors. It is
not primarily to be attributed to the general environ-

[9] See Raymond Pearl, *Studies in Human Longevity* (Baltimore,
Williams and Wilkins, 1924), chapter XI, for a detailed account of
this study.

mental factors connoted by social class distinctions, which are themselves correlated with average energy expenditure in occupation. Before age 40 is attained, it makes no difference in the rate of mortality

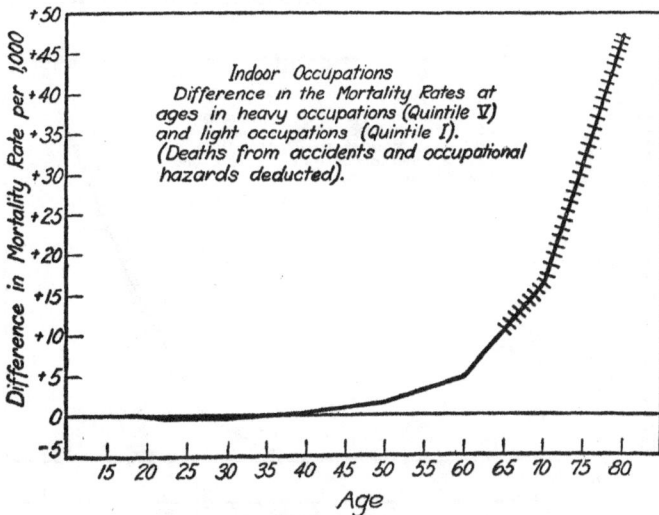

Indoor Occupations
Difference in the Mortality Rates at ages in heavy occupations (Quintile V) and light occupations (Quintile I). (Deaths from accidents and occupational hazards deducted).

FIGURE 14.—Difference between (a) indoor occupations involving the greatest amount of physical exertion (Quintile V) and (b) indoor occupations involving the least amount of physical exertion (Quintile I), in respect of age specific mortality rates. The line is crossed from age 65 on to indicate that its true position is uncertain at advanced ages, because of the meagerness of the data available.

whether the occupation involves light or heavy physical labor. After roughly age 40 to 45 it appears that a man shortens his life, by definite amounts, in proportion as he performs physically heavy labor.

VII

Nothing at all has been discussed about many aspects of the problem of human longevity. These omissions are not to be regarded as consequences of

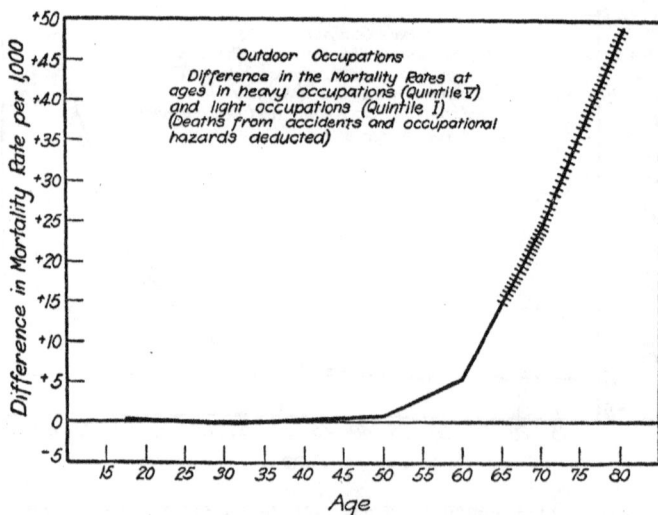

FIGURE 15.—Same as Figure 14, except that it deals with outdoor occupations.

any lack of interest or intrinsic importance in some of the omitted topics. It is mainly a consequence of that profoundly significant fact that a limited space *is* a limited space.

But certain omissions have been deliberate and from principle. Much might have been discussed regarding various theories and speculations about the duration of life that have been put forward in increasing number in recent years. Mostly these have come, directly or indirectly, from consideration of the results of experimental work with lower forms of life. Much of this work has been of fine quality and great intrinsic interest and importance to biology as a science. Some of these experiments have led to highly spectacular success in absolute or relative prolongation of life. For example it has been possible to manipulate seedlings in such a manner as to make them live more than *seven times* as long as they normally would on a given supply of energy and matter as resources for living.[10] Partial or intermittent starvation of various lower animals has led to similar results in the hands of various workers. There is, however, at the present time no smallest reason or justification for even suggesting that results of this sort, and various other sorts in comparable status, have any application whatsoever to human longevity. To insinuate, as some have done in calculated newspaper publicity, that results of this sort might lead in the near future to a startling extension of the human life span is only a bit of naïve professorial *réclame*. When just one single life has been provably prolonged by the application of any such principle its discoverer will not need to advertise. The medical profession will know all about it, and will be testing its possibilities for further extension.

10 S. A. Gould, R. Pearl, T. I. Edwards, and J. R. Miner. On the effects of partial removal of the cotyledons upon the growth and duration of life of canteloup seedlings without exogenous food. *Annals of Botany*, XLVIII, 1934, 575-599.

Again it will have been noted that no advice has been given about how to conduct life so to live long. The reason for this omission is simple. I am not a medical man. It is the proper professional business of medical men to instruct and advise people about healthy and continued living. They have done well at it, and their collective wisdom about it waxes day by day. On the other hand, detached observation suggests that when laymen take on the job, as all too many of them love to do, the results have not been quite universally all that could be desired. Some conspicuous examples could be cited by way of illustration of this point, without having to wander very far geographically. The truth is, as every physician knows, that human life and living are extremely complicated matters, not amenable to simplification by formula or to amelioration by panacea. Really helpful advice about unraveling these complications will come only from the wisdom that grows out of experience and knowledge. The purity of heart and nobility of purpose of bustling "do-gooders" or the ready omniscience of gentry eminent in branches of science *other* than medicine are poor surrogates for the real knowledge and wisdom of the seasoned medical practitioner in the search for longevity.

The literature of longevity is full of advice, recipes, and precepts for the attainment of long life. These precepts touch upon nearly every conceivable aspect of personal physiology and hygiene. Yet it is an odd fact that careful study of our collection of life records of nonagenarians and centenarians leads, as one of the broadest generalizations it is possible to make from them, to the conclusion that these 2,000 and more persons exhibited substantially the same range and degree of variation relative to these various items of personal hygiene as is found among people in general. Some were light eaters, others on the gluttonous side; some used tobacco, others didn't; some drank heavily, others were teetotalers; some slept a lot, others didn't; some had been in robust health all their lives, others had been ailing a great part of the time; and so on. In only one outstanding respect besides great longevity did the group markedly differ from the generality of mankind, on the whole. That is the fact that a vast majority of these extremely longevous folk were of a placid temperament, not given to worry. They had taken life at an even, unhurried pace. In this respect this human material agrees with and confirms a generalization that has emerged from experimental studies on life duration. It is that *the length of life is generally in inverse proportion of the rate of living*. The more rapid the pace of living is, the shorter the time that life endures. This relationship has been shown to exist for a variety of forms, including plants, various lower animals, insects, and men.[11] It is a relation that is obviously in some degree within the power of individual, personal control.

The search for longevity is not ended, though this discussion is. In the view of the biologist the search

[11] For a general discussion of this topic see Raymond Pearl, *The Rate of Living* (New York, Alfred Knopf, 1928), p. 185.

has only just got well under way. A great deal more will be learned, and just possibly we may find out how to lengthen significantly and at will the span of human life, instead of merely increasing its average duration. But if and when this happens the biologist and medical man will probably need to call for the help of the sociologist, the economist and the philosopher to fix over the world, so that it will be better suited for old people to live in than it now is.

VI

MEDICINE AND THE PROGRESS OF CIVILIZATION

BY

REGINALD BURBANK, M.D.

CHAIRMAN, SECTION OF HISTORICAL AND CULTURAL MEDICINE,
THE NEW YORK ACADEMY OF MEDICINE

VI

MEDICINE AND THE PROGRESS OF CIVILIZATION

The origin of the healing art was undoubtedly almost coeval with the advent of man, and began in mystery and superstition. Even to-day, in remote and barbarous regions where the people have not come in contact with civilization, we still find the ancient concept of the healing art. The progress of medicine has always been hindered and encumbered by ignorance and superstition, yet despite this, medical progress has been in the vanguard of civilization. In every great era of the past the doctor has held an important, if not a leading position, until to-day medicine has become such a vital guiding force that modern civilization, as we know it, practically could not exist, were it not for medical initiative.

Early man was little different from the wild beast. When he was injured or diseased, he sought a secluded spot or a cave, either to die or recover. He considered illness due to malevolent, supernatural forces, and was thoroughly imbued with the fear of things he did not understand. He gradually came to feel that it was necessary to placate the evil spirits that caused him to suffer, and this desire led to a belief in the efficacy of magic and the consequent rise of the medicine man. The medicine men of those early days were believed not only to be able to help the sick, but also to bring illness on the well, so they came to be men of considerable importance in primitive communities. How much more perceptive were our early societies! Being more intelligent than the average, the medicine men became priests as well as doctors, and gradually formed a special group. This mingling of religion and healing was a definite manifestation in such high civilizations as Egypt and Babylon.

The function of the medicine man was to frighten evil spirits away, and if the patient had confidence in the ability of the magician, he frequently improved, unless the disease was a fatal one. Such treatment might be considered as the precursor of modern psychotherapy, and was really not dissimilar to the belief produced by some of the cults and fads of to-day. The basis of the treatment was confidence, and confidence has always been the great shield against fear.

In addition to incantations, fetishes made of various animal, vegetable and mineral substances were offered either to placate or drive away the evil spirits. People nibbled at a piece of the vegetable or mineral matter so used and sometimes found an antidote by accident. This gradually led to the discovery of medicines. Most early medicaments used were of no value whatsoever, but some early simples have come down to us and are still esteemed, such as cod liver oil, dried and pulverized dragon bones, furnishing calcium for the prevention of convulsions—these dragon bones were the sun-baked skeletons of prehistoric mammals; colchicum, the poison that Medea brought out of Colchis, still given for gout and arthritis; the juice of the poppy for the sedative action of opium, and many more that could be mentioned, such as sulphur, castor oil, mercury, oxgall and aconite—all dating from before the Christian era.

Most inanimate objects were considered to be imbued with a spirit by primitive peoples, and this spirit was supposed to have power of good or evil: indeed the intoxicating action of fermentation was thought to be due to the "spirit" of the grapes or fruit from which the wine was made, and our word "spirit" was probably so derived.

Plants and herbs thus came to be used for healing and were also used for poisons. Gradually medicine and the black arts came to be associated, not only with magic but with astrology, numerology and colors, particularly in the early civilizations of the Chaldeans, Egyptians, and Babylonians. Nearly all priests of the early civilizations in the East practised astrology and this persisted for thousands of years. The influence exists even to-day, as evidenced by the belief in the influence of the moon, and in the casting of horoscopes. Astrology was practised by physicians up to two hundred years ago. Even Hippocrates, the first scientist in medicine, wrote: "No one should entrust his health and life to one who is not versed in astronomy." Numbers came to be regarded as lucky or unlucky, and treatment was suspended or given according to the numerological portent. Colors had a decided influence. Pink or red medicines were thought to be advantageous for pale people and vice versa. Thus, blood came to be considered a specific for anemia, and so it is.

Prescriptions came into being very early and there are some untranslated ones dating back to the time of Cheops, 3200 B.C. One of the earliest known is a clay tablet from Ur, outlining treatment for a sufferer from rheumatic pain, showing that the arthritic was in need of relief then as he is to-day.

The early Egyptians four to five thousand years back presented a curious mixture of superstition, religion and practical medical and surgical procedure. The priests, who were also the physicians, were restricted to the treatment of diseases with which they were familiar, so you can see there were specialists even in the days of the Pharaohs. The early Chinese physicians were also rigidly restricted, one group for external and one for internal treatments. The old records tell of a man pierced through with an arrow, who went to a doctor; the physician snipped off both ends of the arrow, leaving the rest intact, he told the sufferer to bother him no more but seek an internal specialist for removal of the rest of the weapon.

Medical codes and the restriction of medical practice to those who were qualified occurred early in civilized states. Hammurabi received the medical code from the Sun God, indicating medical restriction among the Babylonians as early as 2250 B.C. In Jewish history we also find divine guidance, and Moses tabulated the first real sanitary code of which we have record. The Mosaic Law was also the most evident example of preventive medicine, but these laws are so mingled with religion that they are seldom thought of as a code of preventive medicine. The priests of all Eastern peoples were associated with such sanitary and preventive measures.

Turning to Greece, which, after all, was the country that influenced the medical and cultural progress of Europe to a greater extent than any other, we find early note of the priests of Asklepios, the Æsculapius of the Romans, mythical son of Apollo, the Sun God and physician. Undoubtedly, Æsculapius was a real man, and was such a good physician that he became the deified hero of medicine, exactly like Hua To' in China. The lovely temples erected to Æsculapius became the early precursors of hospitals and sanatoriums. From his time the emblem of the staff and snake has been used in medicine. His two daughters assisted him in treatment and were also deified. Their names, Hygeia and Panacea, indicate the early belief that since Gods or spirits brought disease, only the Gods could remove or cure it.

The Æsculapian priests did not seek for the cause of a disease, and one of the reasons that the famous Hippocrates was so great is that he was the first definitely to have taken on himself, as a man and not as the representative of a God, the responsibility for cure. The philosophy and ethics of medicine as outlined by Hippocrates persist almost unchanged to the present time, as fundamental as the logic of Aristotle or the unities of the Greek drama. His medical knowledge was drawn largely from the Egyptians, Persians, and East Indians, all of whom had considerable knowledge of drugs and symptoms, so he did not create as much as he coördinated. He was the first to painstakingly record symptoms and physical signs. He took case histories and founded the bedside method which has become the greatest attribute of all real physicians. He first defined and clarified disease and founded the art of diagnosis and prognosis. He dealt with the individual as well as with the disease. His powers of observation were probably unrivaled for nearly two thousand years. His observation "To know is one thing, to believe one knows is another" is the basis of scientific medicine. He wrote "To know is science, but merely to believe one knows is ignorance."

Thus scientific medicine as we know it came into being among the Greeks, and, like all else in that golden period of culture, it reached an apex which was not to be attained again for more than two thousand years. For the first time, common-sense observation, logical deduction, and bedside study were employed in the cure of disease. The highest exemplification of Greek medicine was Hippocrates. The medical codes which he formulated, his study of cases, and his oath of service have become an embodiment of the best in medicine with a persistent influence even to our time.

Along with Hippocrates we find all the great names

of ancient Greece, a civilization which, among the dominant classes, reached a cultural peak that will probably never again be attained. With the decline of this civilization, medicine declined also, but it was not until the sack of Corinth by Rome, 229 B.C., that Greek medicine really fell. The remains of it were carried to Rome where medicine again reached considerable scientific heights with the rise of the Roman Empire. Such great names as Celsus, Dioscorides, Aretæus, and Galen, helped to hold up the Greek tradition. Celsus probably was not a physician but was a wealthy patron of science and literature, who compiled all the medical knowledge of his time. Dioscorides was a Greek army surgeon under Nero, and his *Materia Medica* was a pharmacologic authority for more than fifteen hundred years. Some ninety of his prescriptions are still in use to-day. There were men in those days! Aretæus was another Greek who accurately described pneumonia, tetanus, empyema, the aura of epilepsy, and who also wrote the earliest good accounts of insanity.

Galen was the most skilled physician of his time and formulated the experimental method. He was the undisputed medical authority for the next dozen or more centuries, but he was neither so broad nor so honest as Hippocrates, and while his logic was usually good, his premises were frequently false. He was a theorist with a facile explanation for everything and was a master of dogma rather than of science. His influence, however, became so great that even in Christian times it was considered heresy to doubt him. His system of polypharmacy or shot-gun prescriptions lasted until the Renaissance.

So Rome carried on the Greek tradition but her really great contribution from a medical point of view was sanitation. The Romans built deep sewers to dispose of filth; erected great aqueducts to furnish pure water to the inhabitants and supply the magnificent baths, some of which would accommodate six thousand people. They kept the streets clean and gave the first really extensive application of practical sanitation. They built so well that the sewers and water supply are still in use to-day.

When Rome fell prey to the barbarians both medicine and civilization throughout Europe declined. In the treatment of disease there was again reversion to mystery and magic, which persisted through the Dark Ages and with very few exceptions continued until Arabian culture and medicine were disseminated.

Many causes have been given for the sudden collapse of Roman culture and all had an influence, but one cause is frequently overlooked, namely, the fact that from the Campagna, which Mussolini has lately drained and made arable, malaria gained a foothold in Italy and became a pronounced influence on the physical and mental deterioration of the people.

After the Roman decline, plagues and pestilences came into being, and during the late days of the Empire the practice of medicine deteriorated and lay chiefly in the hands of professional poisoners, courtesans who peddled drugs, and charlatans practicing mystery and magic. During the Dark Ages after the fall of Rome, the priests alone were able to read and write. The imagination of the people was stagnant. There was no impetus to create. Creative spirits were so rare as to be almost non-existent. Authority was vested in the Church and the feudal lord. Monastic medicine came into being. Epidemics decimated the badly drained, pestilential-walled cities. Span of life decreased and infant mortality was appalling. Even as late as five hundred years ago the average life expectancy was but eight years. This shows to what a low ebb medical prevention and practice had fallen, and how few children ever reached maturity. Since then, man's life term has increased approximately fifty years, and medical science has become perhaps the strongest force acting toward human betterment in modern civilization, and this much-vaunted modern civilization is largely built upon medicine in its broader aspects. Our great cities could not exist without medical science.

At low ebb, almost the only vestige of culture that remained of the "grandeur that was Rome" lay in the British Isles and parts of Italy. At the depth of this decadence a new civilization came into being. The Arabs in their frenzy of conquest overwhelmed much of the Mediterranean litoral and but for their defeat at Tour in 732 would probably have conquered all Europe. They built up a high standard of civilization and by the year 900 a cultural height was attained that was not to be approached again until the Renaissance. The Arabs were avid in their search for knowledge, and tolerant of all learning unless it conflicted with their religion. They were responsible for the preservation of the writings of many Greek and Roman physicians, most of which have come down to us through Arabic translations. Prone to disputation, they liked clever logic rather than sound rugged principles such as were advanced by Hippocrates. The sophistic Galen appealed to them far more than did the master of Greek medicine.

The transfer of early medical knowledge to the Arabs came about through contact of the Persians, Arabians, and Jews of Asia Minor with the Greeks of Alexandria, and with the flow of Chinese and Indian knowledge toward the West through the caravan routes from the Orient. The melting pots from which the mingled culture of the East and West was meted out were the Nestorian schools. The first one, founded at Edessa by Nestorius, the patriarch of Constantinople, lasted but a short time, as persecution drove the scholars on to Gande Shapur in Persia on the caravan routes, where the most important group of scholars of this period assembled. This school was destined to be the real birthplace of Arabian medicine and culture. Nestorians and Jews translated the Greek works into Syriac, although it must be admitted that frequently there was definite corruption of sense. In 529 A.D., Justinian the First banished the heathen philosophers from Athens and Alexandria. These scholars traveled eastward and Greek medicine and philosophy became still more firmly established in Persia where the tolerant pagans ruled. At the birth of Mohammed, Gande Shapur was at the height of its fame, and from there the culture and medicine spread to Bagdad.

Arabian physicians and the Nestorians took an active part in the great translating movement into the Arabic. After the Moslem movement, the Caliphs in general were tolerant and offered haven to scholars from all countries. Bagdad rose to great prominence. There were supposed to have been 860 licensed physicians, and numerous hospitals and schools were founded there. After Egypt came under the Caliphate, John the Grammarian rejuvenated the Greek school of medicine at Alexandria, and the Arabians preserved the Greek writings that were not destroyed by the pagan and Christian fanatics of earlier times. The physicians of the time were men of broad cultural background. Rhazes, Haly Abbas, and Avicenna were the outstanding Persian physicians, and the good doctors were acquainted not only with medicine but theology, law, philosophy, astronomy, astrology, music, and chess. Depiction of Arabian physicians carrying the chess board was frequent; if he couldn't play chess, he was not a good physician.

In addition to the knowledge of medicine derived from the Nestorians, the Arabians appropriated many practical points from the sanitary codes of the Jews. They took their astrology from Egypt and the East and, being avid for knowledge, were not hesitant in choosing what they considered the best from all sources. Europe, during this period, was at a very low ebb of culture, and it was not until the *Katib al*

Kullyyat of Averroes that Latin Europe knew or was interested in Aristotle and other Greek philosophers and writers. The Moslem, Geber, acquainted Europe with the alchemy of the East. It was through Albucasis and Avicenna that they knew Galen, the famous Roman physician.

The Chinese influence of the time was chiefly through the culture of Tao, which led to the search for the elixir of life and the philosopher's stone, both impossible to find, but the search for which, through alchemy, led to a considerable degree of chemical knowledge, and distillation, sublimation, calcination and filtration came to be practiced by the Arabs. Nitric acid and *aqua regia,* the solvent which broke down gold, were described by Geber. His *Philosophia Orientalis* did much to influence the thought of that great thirteenth-century scholar, Roger Bacon.

In their travels and conquests, the Arabians found and used many drugs such as ambergris, camphor, cassia, mercury, senna, sandalwood, and so forth. They developed the art of the apothecary and used syrups, alcohol, tragacanth, scented waters, and similar vehicles for the more pleasant taking of medicine, thus greatly improving pharmacy. Many hospitals were founded in the Moslem capitals of Bagdad, Damascus, and Cairo. It is apparently authentic that there were fifty well-supervised hospitals in the city of Cordova alone, about the tenth century. Small hospitals also existed in Europe prior to this time, namely, at Lyons and Merida, but the Arabian hospitals were developed on much more efficient and sanitary lines.

The Arabians were tolerant and humane in the treatment of the insane, and in this were very different from the doctors and priests of Europe. The Moslems founded great libraries where access could be had to all the knowledge of the time. There were 225,000 books at Cordova, and great libraries at Toledo, Seville, and Marcia. The library at Bagdad was noted throughout the civilized world. Arabian civilization at its peak probably surpassed that of Rome. Much of the culture of the western Caliphate was due to constant contact with Bagdad through the peregrinations of the Spanish Jews, and it was partly through the later persecution of the Jews that Islamic culture was spread through Latin Europe. In 1412 they were banished from Spain. The Church at Rome also interdicted Jewish physicians and only lifted the ban toward the end of the fifteenth century. With the exception of Salerno, they were practically excluded from European countries until comparatively modern times, but despite all this, kings, nobles, and popes, utilized their services.

At the peak of Islamic power, the school of Salerno was established near Naples, and there Arabic medicine came in contact with the monastic medicine of Europe. The *Regimen Salernitanum,* the most popular medical book in Europe, was translated into English by Sir John Harrington in Queen Elizabeth's time. Sir John is mentioned as the supposed inventor of the water closet, but we have very good evidence that the flushing toilet was used in Spain under the Caliphate four or five centuries earlier.

The Crusades brought the low culture of Europe in contact with the high Arabic civilization, and during the thirteenth and fourteenth centuries Latin Europe again began to think, but during this time epidemics raged and the black death wiped out half the population. A dancing mania, hysteric dancing, as usual, partly religious, partly sexual, seemed to render mad another half of the remaining population. The schools of Naples, Palermo, Montpellier, and more than a dozen others, drew on the prestige of Salerno to a point where the latter became distinctly second-rate, but it persisted in the shadow of its former grandeur until abolished by Napoleon.

The Arabs actually did not advance medicine to the extent that is generally believed, but they awakened Europe from its lethargy. They did a great deal for pharmacy and were constant searchers for new drugs. These were often brought from great distances, and the search for them led to travel and discovery. Many spices were used in the compounding of medicines, and when these spices and drugs were introduced into Europe they were much sought for and were very expensive, so voyages were made to try to reach the eastern lands of spices by a cheaper and quicker route than the camel caravans of the East. In this way, Arabian medicine became indirectly responsible for the voyages around Africa and even for the discovery of America. Columbus was only sailing

West in the hope of finding an easy approach to the Indies. When he landed, he thought this land was India, and called the natives Indians.

Thus Arabian or Moslem influence awakened Europe and was basically responsible for the Renaissance and the restoration of a cultural civilization. Great names begin to appear as early as the thirteenth century, but it was not until the fifteenth that the full effect of the awakening was seen. Master minds appeared in galaxies, and creative imaginations were again active.

Turbulent men were rulers of Europe at the turn of the sixteenth century. Lorenzo the Magnificent had recently died after being refused absolution at the hands of the implacable Dominican, Savonarola, leaving Florence to revolt and bequeathing the hereditary gout, from which he suffered, to plague the Bourbon dynasty for three hundred years. The gorgeous Borgias were coming to the crest of their influence, and Pope Alexander VI's son, Cæsar, with his *"aut Cæsar aut nihil,"* trying to consolidate temporal power in Italy. Charles V was soon to rule the most extensive realm since the Roman Empire. Francis I was building beautiful palaces and subsidizing art and science in France. Henry VIII was embarking on his career of marriage and intrigue in England. Augustino Barbarigo was Doge of the great maritime state of Venice, which embraced an extensive dominion at that time, and Greece and Italy were little more than its suburbs. Raphael, Brassante, Michelangelo, and Cellini were expanding their careers in art.

With such a background it is small wonder that men of the fifteenth and sixteenth centuries showed truly encyclopedic knowledge. They were examplified by the incomparable Leonardo Da Vinci, who was not only the greatest of painters, but a sculptor, architect, anatomist, musician, poet, engineer, expert on fortification, pioneer in flying, paleontologist, and natural philosopher. No man has ever been more gifted in art and science. It would have been impossible for any man to have accomplished all that he essayed to do. His work and drawings on dissection of the human body undoubtedly stimulated the production of Vesalius' anatomy and may well have been the origin of Servetus' knowledge of aeration of the blood.

Lesser characters in the drama of the Renaissance were numerous. Thomas Linacre, the friend of Erasmus and physician to Henry VIII, was the man responsible for the incorporation of the College of Physicians at London. He was an outstanding character in England.

Jacobus Sylvius, teacher of Vesalius and Servetus at Paris, substituted human bodies for pigs in his dissections, thus restoring medical interest in anatomy.

Fracastorius of Verona wrote *Syphilis sive morbus Gallicus*. This famous poem had as its hero a shepherd called "Syphilis," and from this comes our name for the widespread venereal disease which is so much in the public press these days. This book was very popular and went through many editions. Fracastor was poet, geologist, astronomer, and a physicist as well, and he referred to the magnetic poles of the earth in his writings. As a physician, he wrote on the theory of infection in his *De Contagione*.

Theophrastus Bombastus von Hohenheim Paracelsus, in an overwhelming sense of his own importance, burned the books of Galen and Avicenna before his students, and told them to abandon the ancients. He reformed polypharmacy by making simple extracts and tinctures. He was an alchemist and astrologer as well as physician and surgeon.

François Rabelais was originally a monk but took up medicine and became professor at the University of Montpellier. He translated the aphorisms of Hippocrates, was Curé of Meudon, and was a great exponent of Renaissance humanism. He is perhaps best known as the author of the *Adventures of Gargantua and Pantagruel,* which Voltaire characterized as the foulest vomit that ever drunken monk spewed forth. A large part of his practice seemed to have been confined to venereal diseases.

Luigi Cornaro wrote his *Trattate della vita Sobria* in 1558, probably the best treatise on the simple life and personal hygiene that has ever been written.

Carlo Rinni, at the end of the century, founded modern veterinary medicine.

Timothy Bright, an English physician, wrote a book in 1588 on "arte of shorte, swifte, and secrete writing by character," this being the precursor of

modern shorthand, and the first time brought to the
fore since the time of the Greek heyday.

Despite these and many other great characters of
the times, and the new thought instilled by them,
medicine in the main consisted of blood-letting, herb
doctoring and polypharmacy, and diagnosis was
mostly made by gross examination of the urine. It
seemed as if people spent too much time in fighting to
think much of curing.

Progress continued during the seventeenth century
and many great medical men arose, who, as usual in
those days, were proficient in many branches of learning, and were not restricted to the one-track minds of
so many of our present-day doctors.

Among the great advances of that period of individual scientific endeavor, the seventeenth century,
is that of William Harvey's discovery of the circulation; the actual proof of his belief was due to
mathematical measurements applied to vital phenomena. He was the first man to use this method, and
actually his method of proof was even more important
than the proof itself.

The Chinese philosophy of Wang notes that the
blood cannot but flow continuously like the current
of a river. It may be compared to a circle, without
beginning or end, and all this blood is under the control of the heart. Rabelais, the priest, author, doctor
of the fifteenth century, in the second book treating
the heroic deeds and sayings of the good Pantagruel,

chapter four, also seemed to have a correct idea of the circulatory process.

Michael Servetus, in *Restitutio Christianismi,* 1553, was also on the right track when he noted that the pulmonary circulation passes into the heart after having been mixed with air in the lungs. It seems logical to assume that knowledge of the great advances made in dissection and anatomy by the incomparable Leonardo da Vinci were passed on by word of mouth and became the foundation for this research into the pulmonary circulation. Servetus and his books were both burned by the Church. Columbus, not Christopher, but Realdus, in 1559 published a similar finding on the circulation which may well have been plagiarized from Servetus. But it remained for Harvey to put the theory to experimental proof, and in so doing, institute a new and valuable advance in experimental medicine.

Jenner was another pioneer who was a milestone of progress. He was a quiet, friendly country practitioner of Gloucestershire, who literally founded preventive medicine in the latter part of the eighteenth century, and gave us one of the most valuable of all prophylactic measures: vaccination against smallpox. The idea was not new, having been employed in China for centuries, and the practice of direct inoculation was introduced into England in the early eighteenth century and popularized by Lady Mary Wortley Montague, who wrote and talked about it after her return from Constantinople; but Jenner infected his cases with cowpox and then exposed them to smallpox. These artificially infected cases did not acquire the disease, and some thousands of cases were later proved effectively immunized. Inoculation with, or exposure to smallpox, in subsequent tests, failed to produce the disease. Jenner thus aided in removing one of the world's great scourges. Actually, Louis XV, to my knowledge was the last great personage to die of smallpox. We of to-day can have no realization of what a tremendous scourge smallpox was prior to the nineteenth century. In the *Jesuit Journal* we find an amusing commentary on the remarkable progress of the Jesuit missionaries in converting the Indians, but they note that the devil is jealous of their success and follows them wherever they go, bringing with him an epidemic of smallpox, which decimates the converts after each new advance. This naïve description not only shows the prevalence and danger of smallpox two centuries back, but also demonstrates the extent to which superstition prevailed even among the world's best educated men of the time.

Jenner was reviled and derided in his lifetime, and even to-day we find backward communities that still protest against inoculation. In these areas, small-pox is still endemic.

The proof by Semmelweis that puerperal fever was definitely contagious has not only saved millions of lives, but has been of inestimable value to medicine and the progress of civilization. The fact that this fatal fever was contagious was noted and theorized on by Oliver Wendell Holmes prior to Semmelweis's investigations. The Vienna physician, in 1847, put his belief to the test and forced all the attendants in his obstetrical ward to wash their hands with chloride of lime, upon which female mortality dropped approximately 90 per cent. He thus, without knowing the causative factors, anticipated Pasteur and Koch, but he was laughed at, persecuted, and maligned. Shortly thereafter, he died at Budapest, insane, a thoroughly broken man, again showing how ignorance and prejudice have continuously retarded medical progress, and the progress of civilization. When one considers the appalling maternal mortality of the early days, there can be appreciation of the great influence this concept has had on the increase of population throughout the civilized world.

In 1867, Lord Joseph Lister communicated his success in the prevention of infections by the use of antiseptics. He used carbolic acid and found that with this, wound injuries were no longer dangerous as they did not become infected. This led to the present system of aseptic surgery, which has been the chief factor in the low mortality of modern surgery. Asepsis and anæsthesia together have raised surgery to heights that it could not otherwise have reached, and all this change is in the past hundred years.

The greatest of all advances made in medicine during the nineteenth century, and also the greatest contribution toward our civilized progress that medicine has ever made, was the discovery and study of bacteria as producers of disease.

Bacteria had been known for several centuries before the days of Pasteur. In fact, Varro, about 40 B.C., in *Scriptores Rei Rusticæ* wrote and speculated on "minute organisms which the eye cannot see and which enter the body and cause disease." In 1596, Fracastorius wrote of infection in his *De Contagione*. Athanasius Kircher, the inventor of Eau de Cologne, in his *Scrutinium Pestis,* 1658, noted countless broods of worms not visible to the naked eye, but seen in all putrefying matter under the microscope. He also found the blood of plague patients to be filled with such worms. Leeuwenhoek, 1632-1727, is usually credited with the discovery of the microscope. He really ground better lenses and improved the magnification of an already known instrument, which was almost unquestionably used as early as the thirteenth century by that rare genius, Roger Bacon.

The tireless Hollander, Leeuwenhoek, first gave accurate description of bacterial chains and clumps, and also described bacilli and spirillæ as early as 1683.

Marcus Von Plenciz, in his *Tract Three* on scarlatina, 1762, advanced the idea of a living contagion with a special causative organism for each disease, and he wrote that when the particular seminium verminosum, or germ, of each disease was known, a cure would be possible. This was a splendidly farsighted prophecy, destined to be proved true by Pasteur and Koch.

Pasteur, 1822-95, as a youth, gave promise of being nothing more than a good portrait sketcher and an enthusiastic fisherman. He was graduated at l'École Normale at Paris and developed a decided interest in chemistry. He made many advances in chemistry and disproved the theory of spontaneous generation, but it was not until 1863-65 that he made his far-reaching discovery that partial heat sterilization could be used to kill bacteria without harming taste. This process of pasteurization is now world wide and has been of inestimable importance in the nutrition of children and also in the preservation of food. He discovered the staphylococcus in boils, and the streptococcus pyogenes in puerperal septicemia, confirming the theory of Semmelweis. He accidentally hit upon preventive inoculation, and this led to the use of attenuated viruses. In 1881 he produced a vaccine against anthrax and nearly wiped out the disease in France. In 1885 he treated his first case of rabies with success, and shortly thereafter the Pasteur Institute was opened and became the training school for such men as Roux of diphtheria antitoxin fame; Metchnikoff, who worked on phagocytosis and the lactic acid bacillus; Yersin, Calmette, Chantemasse, and many others.

Despite the honor showered on Pasteur in late life and since his death, he was abused and obstructed in his efforts by the jealousy and ignorance of the physicians of his time. They opposed his work and attempted to stop him from experimental practice because he was a chemist and not a doctor of medicine.

After Pasteur came Koch, who discovered the tubercle bacillus in 1882 and the vibrio of cholera in 1883, thus opening the road to control of two of our most dangerous diseases. Since the time of the two great pioneers, the bacteria or virus of one disease after another has been isolated, and the prophecy of Von Plenciz has been more and more shown to have been extraordinarily clairvoyant.

The great work in constructive and preventive medicine during the nineteenth century was so extensive in scope that only a survey of the highlights is possible. Sanitation was improved. Malaria was controlled. The causative factors in tuberculosis, yellow fever, typhoid, typhus, scarlet fever, syphilis, gonorrhea, and so on, almost ad infinitum, were discovered.

The span of life increased by leaps and bounds. Cities began to increase to unheard-of populations. Refrigeration and pasteurization allowed food to be transported and preserved in the vast metropolitan centers. Huge hospitals arose where difficult surgery became less and less liable to a fatal outcome.

Surgery is a topic that should demand a lengthy commentary, but all we can do now is briefly to outline its origin and early importance, then its decline during the Dark Ages, and the gradual resuscitation after the Renaissance.

The Hindu, Susruta, of about 800 B.C., describes surgery as a "worthy product of heaven," details the need for scrupulous cleanliness of operating room and instruments, and gives the technic of lithotomy—what we now call Cæsarian section, the operation performed for the birth of Julius Cæsar; rhinoplasty, or plastic surgery of the nose; skin grafts, treatment of cataracts, amputations, setting of broken bones, reduction of hernia, and numerous other surgical procedures which we think of as modern.

Greek physicians, perhaps even Hippocrates, visited India and learned some of their medical and surgical practice at this early source of knowledge.

Surgery was esteemed by the Greeks and, to a less extent, by the Romans, but during the Arabian period it fell into disrepute due to the Arabian prejudice against dissection.

During the period of monastic medicine, the Church forbade the use of the knife, and surgery fell into the hands of the barbers, the doctor standing by to give advice but not soiling his hands with the bloody craft. An outstanding exception was Henri de Mondeville, 1260-1320, who urged asceptic treatment of wounds and said that "God did not exhaust all his creative power in making Galen." It was, of course, almost sacrilege to intimate that Galen could have been wrong, so highly was he esteemed.

Guy de Chauliac, 1300-68, was also an erudite surgeon who compiled in a massive book all the existent knowledge of the subject.

After these two, we find no evidence of real progress until Ambroise Paré, 1510-90. He was essentially an army surgeon and served under four kings of France. His pride in his calling was great, and he was respected by friend and foe alike. His saying, inscribed on his statue, *"Je le pansay, Dieu le guerit,"* "I dress the wounds, God cures," became famous and showed his humility. He started as a barber-surgeon in the army at the age of nineteen, and proved to be so expert and kind that he was made surgeon to the king by Henri II. The use of boiling oil as a cautery was discarded by him and cold dressings employed. To him belongs the credit of lifting surgery again to a respected profession.

Little further progress was made in surgery until John Hunter, 1718-83, "the man who refused to stuff Latin and Greek at the University," raised surgery to a true science and made the surgeon a gentleman instead of a servant. He founded modern experimental and surgical pathology. His personal influence was great, but was restricted by a rude and repellent manner. His teachings were spread through his many famous pupils, among whom was the great Jenner. Hunter died, as he often predicted, "at the hands of a rascal who chooses to annoy and tease me"; he was a victim of angina pectoris.

From Hunter's time on, surgery made great strides, and the introduction of asepsis following the antisepsis of Lister and the wider range of procedures permitted by anæsthetics have allowed such extraordinary advances as actually to have added the best part of half a decade to our present life-expectancy.

Forcefully to illustrate the modern progress of surgery, let us take the example of hysterectomy, or removal of the uterus, which, when first practiced in Vienna little more than half a century ago, had a mortality of 96 per cent. An English surgeon insisted on performing the operation on his patients in the last of the preceding century, and all his cases died. The authorities threatened him with prosecution for homicide if he performed the operation again. Finally, unable to resist, he tried it once more and, much to the surprise of his colleagues, the patient lived. At present, this uterine removal holds few terrors for the prospective patient.

To-day, infected wounds and febrile reactions are becoming increasingly rare, and the technic of even the most difficult and dangerous operation has been perfected to a point of comparative safety. Practically all of this progress has been made since the introduction of asepsis and anæsthesia—both, in modern concept, less than a century old.

These great advances in surgery would have been impossible without the use of general anæsthetics by inhalation, crudely employed by the ancients but forgotten for a thousand years. About 800 B.C. the Hindus had the Sammolieni, a method of self anæsthesia through inhalation. In Greek legend, we have the soporific wine that Helen gave Ulysses, and the Hebrews used the *samme de shinta* described in the Talmud, to give relief from pain.

We find the legend that Democedes, the Greek doctor who treated Darius for an injured foot, about 500 B.C., "first eased the pain so as to allow sleep, after which he restored him altogether." In the epic, *Shah Nameh,* there is the legend of obstructed childbirth where the mother is put to sleep and the child taken by operative procedure, the legendary birth of the hero, Jamshid.

Pien Ch'iao and Hua Tao, the deified surgeons of China, were supposed to have used general anæsthetics. They were contemporaries and flourished in the second century A.D.

Dioscorides, in the first century, A.D., used wine of mandragora for anæsthesia in surgical operations, and apparently was conversant with the soporific sponge.

As a matter of pure speculation, it seems probable that the Roman centurion, who offered Christ on the cross a sponge supposedly soaked in vinegar, was not such a heartless brute as might appear. This sponge may well have been a soporific mixture of aconite, dentura, and henbane, knowledge of which had traveled from India and thence to Persia, Greece and Rome. It would seem more likely that a sympathetic centurion, who had knowledge of drugs that would relieve pain, may have attempted to give easement from torture to a Man who was really not considered guilty by his Roman judges. It is possible that the sense may have been garbled in translation. For example, the original Aramaic of the forty-sixth verse of Matthew, twenty-seventh chapter, is "My God, my God, this is my destiny" and not "Why hast Thou forsaken me" as we find it in the King James version. Also, we find in Matthew: "They gave him vinegar to drink mixed with gall," but in Mark is written: "They gave him to drink wine mingled with myrrh."

This may have been the wine of mandragora, a soporific which was often mixed with spices.

Anæsthetics, despite their antiquity, were, like many another bit of knowledge, forgotten and practically unheard of for many centuries. It was not until the time of Simpson, Long, Wells, and Morton, that they were again used for relief of pain in surgical procedure. Crawford Long claimed to be the discoverer of ether anæsthesia, though ether was known as early as the sixteenth century, and performed the first operation on a patient under its influence in March, 1842. Horace Wells first used nitrous oxide gas as an anæsthetic in dentistry in 1844. A fatal result caused him to withdraw from practice, and he eventually committed suicide. William Morton, a dentist in Charlton, Massachusetts, used ether to produce anæsthesia for operations in 1846. Sir James Simpson used chloroform as an anæsthetic in midwifery about the same time. The terms "anæsthesia" and "anæsthetic" were both introduced by our own Oliver Wendell Holmes, coined from the Greek *an,* without or not, and *æsthesis,* feeling; another medical contribution from the brilliant doctor who is usually thought of as a master of literature, not of medicine.

During the nineteenth century, many great advances were made in constructive medicine. Philippe Pinel, 1755-1826, was the first modern who attempted to improve the condition of the insane. He placed the mentally incompetent in hospitals and tried to classify the patients according to the character of their mental diseases. He was really the first since the days of the Arabs to treat the insane by gentle means. He instituted physical labor instead of corporal punishment. This work marked a definite epoch in the study of psychiatry. Since his time, we all know of the great effort made to treat the insane in a humane manner and try and bring a certain per cent of these unfortunates back to useful lives. During the past two decades, numerous hospitals have been built by the state to take care of the feeble-minded and attempt reconstruction by adapting them to their environments.

During the Napoleonic Wars, a French army surgeon by the name of Dominique Jean Larrey instituted so-called "flying ambulances," which permitted quick care of the wounded after their injuries and prevented innumerable deaths from infection from wounds contaminated on the field of battle. His work led to the formation of the ambulance corps as it is known to-day. Larrey was a remarkable surgeon with distinctly modern ideas. He was an indefatigable worker and performed as many as two hundred operations in the course of a single day.

René Theophile Hyacinthe Laënnec discovered the stethoscope and published his classical treatise on auscultation in 1819. Thanks to him we have been able to pursue more accurate investigations of the chest. His work permitted a greatly enlarged field of study in tuberculosis. Laënnic died a young man of forty-five from the very disease that his investigations made easy of early diagnosis. Since his time, continued investigations have led to successful treatment of tuberculosis and it is no longer the dreaded disease that it was a century ago.

William Beaumont, another army surgeon, published in 1833 his famous experiments and observations on a case of accidental gastric fistula and founded our modern concept of dietetic tables and scales. He studied on the human what Pavlov in Russia proved on dogs three-quarters of a century later, and his work led to investigations responsible for a great share of our knowledge of gastric function and intestinal digestion.

Galvani, Volta, and Franklin paved the way for the electrical researches that made electricity the servant of mankind that it has now become. Leaving aside the medical field and the great advances in physiotherapy that their work permitted, the benefit to civilization of the result of their discoveries is almost inestimable, and electricity in its multiform uses has become such an accepted adjunct to our civilized life that we take its benefits for granted and scarcely consider its tremendous importance.

Sternberg, Laveran and Munson, in their work on malaria, have made it possible gradually to eradicate one of the world's great scourges. Before their time, no one knew how the disease was spread, but after the mosquito was proved to be the malarial carrier, prevention became possible, resulting in the preservation of the health of millions.

Walter Reed, James Carroll, Jesse Lazear and Agramonte were the heroes of the yellow fever experiments which cost Lazear his life. They proved that yellow fever was caused by the bite of an infected mosquito. The method of proof was an heroic one as they allowed themselves to be bitten by mosquitoes suspected of carrying the disease. Their work led to the almost complete extermination of this deadly disease in many areas, perhaps the most spectacular being Havana and Panama, where Gorgas practically rendered yellow fever non-existent.

Alexander Graham Bell, a professor of physiology in Boston, who came to this country from Canada, was the man whose inventive genius made possible our present system of verbal communication, which has practically annihilated space. His medical work was of little significance, but the invention of the telephone, for which he was responsible, brought about a revolution in communication.

Fritz Schaudinn discovered that the spirocheta pallida was the causative organism in syphilis, and the present treatment by mercury, arsenic, and bismuth, is gradually decreasing the ravages of this dread venereal disease. No longer do we see great syphilitic ulcerations, or patients with sunken noses and unsightly scars. Also, this disease has now been driven into the open and the present publicity drive against the scourge of syphilis should do much to eradicate it in the next few generations.

Roentgen, discoverer of the X-ray, made it possible to see into and through the human body, and has rendered possible diagnosis that could not have been made prior to his time.

During the past fifty years, we have seen rabies, typhoid, typhus, cholera, dysentery, and diphtheria practically eradicated in civilized states. Syphilis and tuberculosis have been shown to be curable and have lost much of their terror. Diabetes and pernicious anemia are both controllable, thanks to the discovery of insulin by Banting and the application of liver extract by Minot and Murphy.

We are gradually learning to subdue the ravages of that greatest of all incapacitators, arthritis, and this despite the fact that as yet no adequate provision is made for its treatment in the majority of our great modern hospitals.

Cancer, unfortunately, still retains its terror, with early surgery and radium or X-ray as the only measures which can be depended on to reduce its ravages. Progress has been scant in this field, despite the fact that millions have been spent in research.

The medical advances which we have quoted, and myriads of others which space forbids even mentioning, have prolonged the span of life and allowed enormous numbers, who would otherwise have died, to live on to ripe old age. Child mortality has decreased to an astounding degree. Sanitation, preservation of food, and quick communication have rendered possible our huge modern cities with their ever mounting populations. Modern surgery has permitted countless thousands to live, who, in the old days, would have died without the benefit of operative procedure.

The result has been an enormous increase in the world's population during the past hundred years, and the keeping alive of innumerable unfit, many of whom have become a distinct economic problem for society and the state. In the present world unrest, where mounting populations continuously create new economic problems, medicine may almost seem to be defeating its own ends and making life more difficult for the majority, but certainly had it not been for the doctor and his works, modern civilization, as we know it, would not and could not exist.

VII

X-RAY WITHIN THE MEMORY OF MAN

BY

LEWIS GREGORY COLE, M.D.

CONSULTING ROENTGENOLOGIST, FIFTH AVENUE HOSPITAL

VII

X-RAY WITHIN THE MEMORY OF MAN

WHEN asked by the president of the Academy, Dr. James Alexander Miller, to discuss the early history of X-Ray, I said I preferred to discuss "X-Ray Within the Memory of Man," specifically within the memory of this old man, that is what I propose to do. As these oft-told yarns were assembled, they seemed to record an overwhelming amount of personal activity, and so they do. In those early days there were three-score, or possibly three-score and ten of these early X-ray workers who were having exactly the same experiences as I herein relate, in the various fields of X-ray development. And I would that those few who are left of the early pioneer workers would narrate these personal instances for permanent record, as I am doing.

Like many other discoveries of far-reaching importance, X-ray was discovered almost by accident. Late in November, 1895, William Konrad Roentgen announced that he had discovered X-ray while working with a vacuum tube designed by Crooke. Undoubtedly Crooke and many other scientists had already obtained X-rays from similar tubes without recognizing their significance or even their existence. They were like children at a treasure hunt, where each searches diligently until one of them says, "Here it is. I have found it." Roentgen deserves more credit for his fortitude in withholding the announcement until he had made thorough investigation of this new power than he does for the actual discovery of the X-ray.

When this startling announcement was finally made, the result was electrifying. Apparently an unbelievable number of people had been working along similar lines, so that within a short time of Roentgen's announcement some variety of X-ray examination was being made in many parts of the world. These investigators included all ranks of scientists from the great Edison down to many backwoods would-be researchers who had an inclination for investigation but no adequate laboratory apparatus. One scientist in the latter category constructed an X-ray tube from the chimney of a kerosene lamp, and with this primitive apparatus made an X-ray of a mouse. I later saw the lamp chimney X-ray tube and the roentgenogram.

Roentgen's discovery had indeed caused a furor in the world of science. Like other great discoverers, he did not realize the full implications of what he had done. He was a pure scientist, and in fact he seemed to resent the application of the X-ray to utilitarian purposes, or even for roentgenologic diagnosis. Fortunately, however, Roentgen's distaste for these aspects of his discovery had little effect upon the more practical scientists who were eager to apply this new energy to the problem of medical diagnosis.

As might be expected, Thomas Edison, and his co-worker, Clarence Dally, were well in the vanguard of experimentation and in the construction of new apparatus. Dally worked incessantly investigating this new field of radiation. Since neither he nor anybody else at that time knew of the dangers of X-ray, it is no wonder that he was the first martyr to the new science. The fact that he died so soon after is testimony to the prodigious amount of work he did in a short time. Unfortunately for the science of roentgenology, Edison was so shocked by the death of his friend and beloved co-worker that he immediately ceased his investigations.

Many workers felt that Dally's death was not caused by the X-ray, but shortly afterwards in Rochester, New York, a man by the name of Weigal met a similar fate. X-ray had claimed its second victim. This established beyond any question that X-ray had malignant powers. The problem of harnessing these forces to serve rather than to destroy was yet to be solved.

In the early part of this century X-ray was one of the youngest in the family of medical specialties. According to George Johnson, the noted wit of the American Roentgen Ray Society, the baby of the family—nicknamed X-ray and rechristened roentgenology—was born with a breech presentation, brought into the world by a midwife, and wet-nursed by janitors, elevator boys, electricians, apothecaries, photographers, and even steam-fitters. Black art and charlatanism were only a few of the names she was called, but, like Topsy she just "growed" in spite of all obstacles, and became an important member of the family of medical specialties.

Philadelphia had a group of active roentgenologists such as Leonard, Kassabian, Pfhaler, Pancoast, and others, who made their city a Mecca for all roentgenologists. Boston, too, had its group of early workers, stimulated especially by the work of Williams, Dodd, and Rollins, a dentist who wrote a book on technic that was really quite remarkable. Williams very early recommended X-ray for gastro-intestinal examinations, and advocated a mixture of bismuth and gruel as an opaque media. His recommendations attracted little attention in this country, except from his admiring young medical student, Walter Cannon, whose goose and cat are now famous throughout the world. Five years later Reider, either with or without knowledge of Williams' work, recommended the identical mixture of bismuth and gruel, which became known as the Reider meal. As soon as this announcement was made by Reider and the recommendation came from Germany, it was adopted in this country by Americans, especially German-American roentgenologists, who sang its praises. In 1905, Hulst returned from Munich, where he had seen the work of Reider, and showed a series of roentgenograms using the so-called Reider meal at the Congress of the American Roentgen Ray Society in Baltimore in 1905.

As a matter of fact Hemmeter of Baltimore claimed priority in making the first gastro-intestinal examination by the use of an opaque media in the stomach.

There was, and still is, some controversy as to whether his first examination by this method at the Normal School in Baltimore preceded an announcement of the method by a German named Wolff. There is some evidence to show that Hemmeter's manuscript was in the hands of a publisher before Wolff's announcement was made. At any rate, it was an almost simultaneous discovery.

The pioneer roentgenologists worked in groups. At least they met regularly in the evenings to discuss their work, their methods, and especially to discuss ways of improving apparatus. A group of these early workers in the Middle West, composed of Hickey, Van Zwallen, Dachtler, Lang, Crane, and Hulst, were extremely active in the development of roentgenology in Ohio, Michigan, and Indiana. Stover and Childs of Denver carried the work farther west, and Stover carried it even to the coast and to Hawaii.

George Johnson of Pittsburgh devoted much of his time toward integrating these small local groups into one large association of roentgenologists who met once or twice a year to exchange ideas. This association soon developed into the American Roentgen Ray Society. Boggs, also of Pittsburgh, was one of the early enthusiastic roentgen therapists. Gray of Richmond, and a little later Samuels of New Orleans represented the Southern group of roentgenologists.

Space does not permit enumerating these pioneer roentgenologists and recounting their achievements. Instead I shall recommend the book written by Percy Brown of Boston. Like many of the courageous pioneers, he is himself a great sufferer from the effects of X-ray. Thus he was inspired to write a book on the achievements of other roentgenologic martyrs, which tells their stories much better than I could hope to do in this brief discussion.

Baetjer was the outstanding man in Baltimore in those early days, and his work on the diagnosis of bone lesions is a classic that will be an everlasting monument to his memory. I consider Caldwell, Snook, Waite, and Dachler, the outstanding men in this country in the development of X-ray apparatus and in the perfection of X-ray technic in those early days. Considerably later, Professor Schearer of Cornell entered the field, and was a great coördinator between the ultra-scientific physicists and the practical roentgenologists.

In our own city of New York, Caldwell, Dickson, Dieffenboch, Piffard, Basser, Taussey, Beck, Holding, and myself, were the early workers, and very soon Law, Jaches, Imboden, McKee, and Remer, entered the field.

But I believe that Caldwell was the first X-ray specialist in New York. Trained as an electrical engineer, he was one of the multitude of scientists who sensed the approach of the era of irradiation long before it arrived. At first he was more interested in the long wave, which eventually developed into radio, but he soon embarked on an active career in this new short-wave energy, X-ray. His electrical training led him to adopt the coil, and soon he constructed a larger coil for the production of X-ray. Then he developed the electrolytic interruptor which bears his name, and which will be his memorial in scientific history. Although not yet a doctor, he opened an office in the back room of Ford's Instrument Store, located, if I remember correctly, on Fifth Avenue at Twenty-eighth or Twenty-ninth Street. There he began as New York's first specialist in the application of X-ray to the practice of medicine. It is doubtful if at that time he had any idea of the importance of his step, for a short time later he tried to discourage me from entering the field by telling me that I should not abandon my surgical career, and also that there was not room in New York for more than one X-ray man. His advice, I am certain, was sincere and not influenced by any fear of competition, because many others told me the same thing. George Creevey, one of my fellow interns at Roosevelt Hospital, argued with me into the wee small hours trying to dissuade me from giving up a life career as a surgeon for what he called "medical photography."

I well remember the first time I heard the word *X-ray*. During my second year as student at P & S, my brother-in-law one morning pushed the *Times* across the breakfast table. "Lew, what do you think of this? Some man in Germany has discovered a light with which you can see through people." I glanced at the article, and with the assurance of a young medical student, I replied, "Why, there's nothing to it. Only the other day one of my professors at the college told us that any announcement made to the newspapers was likely to be a fake, that any announcement of real medical advancement was made to the medical journals first."

With the rest of the world, I laughed at the newspaper cartoons depicting the bones of a presumably lovely girl sitting on the bony lap of her escort's skeleton. My next recollection of the X-ray was seeing the roentgenogram of Professor Weir's hand. We all then said, as novices still say, "Oh, look at his ring! It doesn't even touch his hand."

My first serious introduction to the X-ray was during my internship at Roosevelt Hospital. That was in 1898 and 1899. McBurney was keeping the rest of the surgical staff busy all day in the operating room, so the fractures in the accident room fell to my lot—besides nobody else wanted them anyway. About a year of this experience gave me confidence in my ability to treat fractures. One day there came in a compound fracture of both bones of the leg, and I was permitted to treat it with open operation. I succeeded in slipping the ends of the bones in such perfect apposition that they promptly united. Clinically the result was so good as to attract some attention.

Grimshaw, then apothecary and assistant superintendent of the hospital, suggested that I take the patient down to the Hudson Street Hospital, where they had just installed a new X-ray apparatus. As far as we knew it was the only one in the city at that time. With old Billyhorse, and Heinz, the Dutch ambulance driver, we took the patient down-town. We entered the basement, avoiding steam pipes overhead and electric wires all around, until we found the engine room, where the X-ray apparatus was set up just above the engineer's work-bench, which served as the X-ray table. I said I would wait for the X-rays to be developed, but the engineer who was also the X-ray man said, "Oh, no. We have to wait until it is dark enough to develop them right here on the work-bench. You see, we haven't any darkroom."

The next morning I returned, eager to see the result. What I saw in the X-ray film gave me the shock of my life. While the ends of the bones showed remarkably good position, the bones themselves were bowed backwards until they formed a semicircle. I was disgusted with this new-fangled method of diagnosing fractures. Clinically we knew that the ends of the bones were in good apposition, so this X-ray was obviously in error. Nevertheless, on my way back to the hospital I was strongly tempted to hurl the X-rays out the window of the Ninth Avenue elevated train or to drop them into an ash-can rather than show them to my colleagues, who, as I well knew, would ride me unmercifully. This riding I got good and plenty, but perhaps it was a good thing, for it prompted me to investigate the use of X-ray in the treatment of fractures.

No X-ray machine was available for my work, so I constructed a crude apparatus of my own. I put an incandescent lamp into a shoe-box, in which I had punched a hole. This served as an X-ray tube. Of course this contraption would not photograph bones with flesh on them, so from the dissecting room I obtained some bones without flesh, which I fractured for my experiments. By moving the bones, the light, and the paper on which I traced the shadow, into different positions, I proved to my own satisfaction that we could get almost any distortion in the X-ray. I began to write a paper entitled "Skiographic Errors in the Treatment of Fractures." Skiogram was the word then used for X-ray.

It required some eight or ten months to complete the experiments, and about that time an X-ray machine was installed at Roosevelt Hospital. It was operated by Dr. Percy Turnure, in fact I am not sure but what he gave the machine to the hospital. Convinced of skiographic errors in fractures, day after day I watched Dr. Turnure make examinations of various bones. To my astonishment, I saw that in X-rays of real fractures, with relatively uniform positions of tube, plate, and part, these errors did not occur. A little reluctantly, I was converted, and though I finished the article and kept the name "Skiographic Errors in the Treatment of Fractures," I added "And How They Can Be Prevented."

Soon after the shoe-box experiments, Van Allen of Springfield, one of the early workers in roentgenology, and the David Harum of X-ray, wanted to buy a new coil to replace his old Kincaid coil. He went to the Cornell Medical School to seek the advice of their roentgenologist, Arthur Holding. Dr. Holding referred him to "that young fellow up at Roosevelt Hospital." Dr. Holding told him that according to what he had heard, this young fellow had cut off the ends of the primary of an old Willyoung coil, and with this reconstructed apparatus was able to get fairly good roentgenograms, especially in combination with an electrolytic interruptor, which it was reported that he tuned by ear. The story of Van Allen's purchase is full of human interest, and its influence on X-ray history was considerable.

What Holding had heard was essentially correct. With this old, discarded, sawed-off, hammered-down coil, in combination with an electrolytic interruptor and a thoroughly seasoned Gunderloch tube, we had obtained roentgenograms which showed remarkable detail—even the hips, pelvis, and lumbar spine were fairly clear.

Professor Weir, to whom I have previously referred, had seen at a Philadelphia meeting some X-rays made by Leonard which showed kidney stones. He returned full of enthusiasm and eager to get me to make similar roentgenograms. I well remember my remark, "I think, as a roentgenologist, we would do well to limit our examinations to bullets and bones." But Weir was persistent in his quiet way, and finally he persuaded me to get out all our X-rays of the lumbar spine. He remarked that these showed much more detail than those in which he had seen the kidney stones. Holding them up to the north light (we had no light-box in those days), he called my attention to areas of diminished density on each side of the lumbar spine, and below these a pyramidal shadow whose base seemed to be at the crest of the ilium. He pointed out to me, "Why isn't this pyramidal shadow the psoas muscle on each side, and these less distinct shadows above look like the kidneys. Aren't they the shape of the kidneys?" And much to my surprise I observed that they were.

With much enthusiasm on his part and some on mine, we then attempted to make X-ray examinations of patients suspected of having kidney stones. By compressing the parts, we showed clearly that one of these patients had a stone in the lower end of the ureter. Unfortunately for Weir, this was not one of his cases; it was William T. Bull's, who was not at all enthusiastic about the X-ray. He based his diagnosis on clinical evidence of stone in the ureter, and he paid little attention to what the X-ray showed or didn't show.

Naturally we were intensely interested in the operation on this patient. When Bull cut down on the ureter near the bladder, there was no stone to be found. He palpated the ureter and still could not find a stone. He then made a small slit in the ureter above, and passed a flexible catheter into the bladder without encountering any obstruction. Those of you who remember Bull can well picture his state of mind. He was like his proverbial namesake in the china shop. With the assurance which only ignorance can give, I insisted that there must be a stone in the ureter. Had I not proved it with my X-ray? Dame Fortune smiled on me that day, for eventually they found a stone the size of a pea, located in a pouch protruding from the ureter in such a way as not to obstruct its lumen. There was some controversy as to whether it was a urinary calculus or a gland that was adherent to the ureter. Dame Fortune smiled on me again, for on section it proved to be a stone composed of urates.

Stones located in the kidney proper were a different problem, however. Since the kidney moves with respiration, our exposures of a minute and a half yielded such blurred negatives that we could not determine with certainty the presence of stones, especially small, single stones. We then attempted to adjust the apparatus so that we could make exposures in thirty seconds, while the patient held his breath. We did this with what we called an old seasoned gas tube and just the proper hum to the electrolytic interruptor. But I think the most important thing was to get a patient who was thin enough to be squeezed down tightly. These were the days before kilovolt meters were ever heard of and even long before the milliamperemeter was used. In those days the making of an X-ray was an art, not a science.

Leonard considered the X-ray only an adjunct in the diagnosis of kidney stone, and whether the stones showed or didn't show had no influence on whether the surgeon would operate on the patient for a kidney stone.

At the invitation of Dr. Keyes I presented a paper before the Bellevue Alumni Association on the diagnosis of kidney stones, and soon afterwards one before a combined meeting of the American Urological Society and the American Obstetrical Society in Baltimore. At that time I maintained that the diagnosis of kidney stone should be based primarily on the roentgenograms, and that the patient should not be operated upon for kidney stones when the X-ray was negative, unless, of course, the symptoms were overwhelmingly characteristic. This contention was kindly accepted by the two societies, but shortly after this, when I made a similar statement before one of the sections of the American Medical Association, it caused so much resentment that I was not allowed to finish the discussion.

Shortly after this, Caldwell, whom I have already mentioned, did his famous work on the diagnosis of frontal and accessory sinus diseases. Caldwell, always modest, was especially diffident because he had not yet received his medical degree. As a result, the nose and throat men with whom he had worked in this series of cases "ran off with the bone." The only credit which Caldwell received from this monumental work was given to him by his colleagues in the field of roentgenology. They immortalized him by giving his name to the 23-degree position for making roentgenograms of the frontal sinus.

In my X-rays of the chest for fractured ribs I had noticed that in some cases there showed areas of increased density which seemed to be in the lungs. At this time, after the episode with Weir and the kidney shadows, we were acutely "soft tissue conscious." Some of these shadows which showed in X-rays of the thorax were relatively dense and as large as a lemon, whereas others had a mottled appearance. Most of them appeared in the upper part of the lung. The question as to what caused these shadows thrust

itself upon us. Clinical history indicated that many
of these patients had a cough, some loss of weight,
and shortly it developed that most of them had some
kind of lung trouble. It then dawned upon us that
the increased density in the lung might possibly be
tuberculosis of the lung.

Enthusiastic about the possibilities of X-ray as a
method of diagnosis of pulmonary tuberculosis, I
wanted to get uncut specimens of tuberculous lungs,
so that I could inflate these lungs and make X-ray
examinations outside of the body. I went to a pathologist at my own college, a man who had been a friend
of the family for many years. I told him of my observations of increased lung density and of the other
work we had done in soft tissues, and asked him if
he could let me have specimens of tuberculous lungs
for my experiments. Such specimens lay there on a
tray within my reach, and I walked over to pick them
up, saying that this was exactly what I wanted. He
took me by the shoulder, turned me around, looked
me squarely in the eye, and said, "Young man, there
is nothing to this X-ray diagnosis. It is nothing more
or less than black art, and any one who attempts to
use it is a charlatan. Because of my respect for your
family, I not only will not give you those lungs, but
I will do everything in my power to prevent you
from getting them elsewhere." Surprised and stunned,
I went to the door, opened it, and walked down four
flights of winding stairs, acutely conscious of the stern
figure standing at the open door watching my retreat.
The irony of it was that this very pathologist died

of tuberculosis some time after that; he probably had it at the time. If his lesion had been recognized by this method which we were trying to establish, undoubtedly his life would have been prolonged and perhaps he would have lived to a ripe old age.

Undaunted by this rebuff, I went to Ewing, the recently appointed pathologist at Cornell. He was intensely interested in my problem, but since he had few autopsies of tuberculous patients, he sent me to Dr. Norris and Dr. Schultz, who were pathologists at Bellevue Hospital. They were enthusiastic about my experiment, and not only supplied me with the specimens I needed, but allowed me to set up an X-ray apparatus in the old morgue at the foot of Twenty-sixth Street. The new one, I believe, they call a "mortuary." Harry Waite, of Waite and Bartlett, loaned me the apparatus, and with it I made many roentgenograms of inflated lungs. Down in the old morgue I got my first real taste for research work, and my appetite for it has never been sated.

As soon as the inflated lungs had been X-rayed they were sliced as one would slice liver. Then each slice was laid out on a slab, examined, palpated, and the surface wiped with the back of a knife so that we could more accurately observe pathological findings. The grosser lesions which had been observed in the roentgenograms were confirmed in the cut sections. Many of the X-rays, however, showed small isolated areas of density which were in the middle of the slice, and so were not visible on either cut surface. Ewing removed these areas, examined them microscopically, and confirmed the X-ray diagnosis by stating that they were small, firm, isolated tubercles. Then I maintained that the diagnosis of pulmonary tuberculosis could be made by X-ray recognition of small, isolated, miliary tubercles.

The roentgenograms which I had made in this work, together with roentgenograms of clinical cases, obtained largely from the Vanderbilt Clinic through the courtesy of Dr. Austin Riggs, were assembled in an exhibit which was shown at the International Congress of Tuberculosis in Washington, in the spring of 1907. Delafield and Pruden's *Pathology of Tuberculosis* provided most of the descriptive captions for the exhibit. Delafield's interest was aroused, and he spent much time in going over the exhibit with me. LeWald says that his interest in X-ray dates from that day at the International Congress when he heard Delafield and me discuss the possibilities of X-ray in the diagnosis of pulmonary tuberculosis.

Stimulated perhaps by Delafield's flattering interest, I stuck closer than ever to his classification of pulmonary tuberculosis. A more intensive study of these anatomic-clinical roentgenograms and the attempt to correlate my X-ray findings with Delafield's pathologic findings, led to an article presented at the meeting of the American Roentgen Ray Society in September, 1907. This article advocating X-ray as the method of diagnosing pulmonary tuberculosis started a cyclonic controversy. The Society immediately went into executive session to determine whether they should publish such a radical article, fearing that it might reflect discredit upon their national society. I have always been grateful to Crane for coming to my rescue.

This article was first published in the *Transactions of the American Roentgen Ray Society* and later in the *American Journal of the Medical Sciences* in July, 1910. The controversy caused by this article lasted nearly a decade. I can only say that, thirty years later, I have nothing to add to and nothing to retract from the original article as it was published in the *American Journal of Medical Sciences* to which Lawrason Brown eventually paid a great compliment.

In 1909 our interest shifted to the problem of gastro-intestinal diagnosis by X-ray. For more than five years X-ray had been used on the continent, and to some extent in this country, for the study of gastro-intestinal lesions. The "continental" or "indirect method" was based on what were termed "symptom complices." That is, roentgenological evidence of the way in which the stomach functioned was combined with evidence gained from clinical history, physical examination, and gastric analysis. In contrast to this method there was developed, largely in this country, what we called the "American" or "direct method." In this method we diagnosed gastro-intestinal pathologic lesions directly by use of X-ray, showing in our roentgenograms the manner in which a cancer protruded into the lumen of the stomach or the manner in which an ulcer formed a crater or niche which projected beyond the lumen of the stomach. For some time there was considerable rivalry between the two methods.

When I first saw an X-ray of the stomach after an opaque meal had been ingested, I felt that it was not quite "cricket" to aid the X-ray diagnosis by putting something of increased density into the intestinal tract so that it could be more easily visualized. It seemed to me that this was like retouching the negative. I thought that the X-ray technic should be improved so that it would not be necessary to use these opaque media to show the stomach and bowels.

In 1906 "Roentgenograms of the Normal Stomach" was the title of Hulst's presidential address at the Niagara meeting of the American Roentgen Ray Society. In this address Hulst made his famous remark, "Show me a Venus de Milo and I will show you a normal stomach." Since the roentgenograms which he showed us were made with a coil and without an intensifying screen, the time required for exposure was so long that the movement of the stomach caused considerable blurring. Therefore they were of little value for the diagnosis of gastro-intestinal lesions. Their chief value was in showing that the size, shape, and position of the stomach were actually not as pictured in the anatomy texts of that time or even in those of to-day. Then there resulted an epidemic of erroneous diagnosis of prolapsed stomach, many of which were operated upon and strung up by some kind of surgery.

At that same meeting Snook presented data on the type of high tension energy that was developed from the coil with various types of interruptors. From this data he later developed a transformer with a rectifying switch which enabled us to make X-rays with a much shorter exposure. A year or two later the advent of the intensifying screen enabled us to make X-rays of the gastro-intestinal tract so rapidly that blurring due to movement was eliminated.

Thus for the first time we were able to recognize lesions of the stomach which protruded into the lumen or rendered the stomach wall less pliable. I well remember my excitement at my first diagnosis of carcinoma of the stomach. The patient was a society woman, and, feeling no symptoms, she was bored with the examination. When I asked her to come back so that I could make a six-hour plate, she said that she couldn't possibly spare the time, for she was going to a party where they were going to play a new game called "auction." She said it was something like whist. This fairly well establishes the time. Within a week she was operated upon, but she never did learn to play "auction."

After this diagnosis of carcinoma we rapidly began to make diagnoses of ulcers of the stomach, gallbladder diseases, cancers of the colon, and a little later, diverticuli of the colon and of the duodenum. All this occurred within a decade. First "bullets and bones," then kidney stones, infection of the frontal and maxillary sinuses, tuberculosis of the lungs, gastro-intestinal disorders of all kinds—all these disclosed their secrets to the X-ray within the memory of man.

When you and I are long since gone, and when missions and churches and galleries and libraries have been destroyed, and historical and scientific books have been burned by political leaders in order that others may be written to record their own power and glory, the history of medicine of the twentieth century will be written. It may run something like this, provided of course there are any intellectuals left to write it or any one sufficiently intellectual to wish to read it. The historian of the future will say, "More than a hundred years ago, just at the end of the nineteenth century, a new manifestation of energy was discovered by a man named Roentgen. This energy was an unknown factor in the field of physics, so he termed it 'X' to which the word 'ray' was soon added. Shortly after this Pierre Curie and his wife discovered radium, an element emanating a similar manifestation of energy. This new element gave forth energy that was almost perpetual motion." This historian, some sixty years hence, at the beginning of the twenty-first century, will go on to say, "The first milligram of radium made by the Curies is giving off as much energy to-day as it did the day it was first discovered.

"At about the same time there was developed a radiant energy by which the sound of the human voice was transmitted to the very ends of the earth, literally from pole to pole. At first these radiant energies of the twentieth century, like the machines of the nineteenth century, were harnessed and used for man's benefit. Just at the beginning of the twentieth century, when man had reached the peak of western civilization, the application of X-ray to the practice of medicine had a more profound influence on medicine than any other factor recorded in the whole history of medicine. To be sure, the discovery of ether made surgery practical; Pasteur's discovery made surgery safe; but the discovery of X-ray made it possible to determine when to operate and when not to operate. It was applicable both as a diagnostic and as a therapeutic agent in practically all fields of medicine.

"Although the application of X-ray to medical diagnosis was seemingly slow in getting started it developed with extreme rapidity when it did get started. The diagnosis of 'bullets and bones,' kidney stones, pulmonary tuberculosis, frontal and accessory sinus diseases, mastoid, cancers of the stomach, ulcers of the stomach, post-pyloric ulcers, and the diagnosis of other lesions of the entire gastro-intestinal tract were developed within a single decade, that is, from 1905 to 1915."

The historian will continue to say, "Those must have been grand and glorious days, and what a thrill it must have been to have lived in that time and to have played some minor part in that drama of life and death at the birth of X-ray diagnosis.

"Strange as it may seem, there were only a few developments in the application of X-ray to the practice of medicine after the beginning of the first World War. Gall bladder dyed by Graham? Yes. Air in the ventricles by Dante? Yes. Lipodol in the lungs? Yes. But these were only as a few drops in the bucket when compared with the developments of X-ray between 1905 and 1915.

"Not all the developments of X-ray made during this short period of time were universally used at that time, but they were known to and used by a few roentgenologists, and one of the blessings of the first World War was that hundreds of doctors were trained in the medical corps to use the X-ray and to apply this method of diagnosis to all branches of medicine. When the war was over, these men, well trained in roentgenology, were free to apply their skill in civil practice in all parts of the world. Such a large number of roentgenologists would never have had such an intensive training in such a short period of time if it had not been for the first World War. Can you imagine the surgeon searching for bullets or shrapnel in the mangled bodies of the victims of the first World War without the use of X-ray, though they did have ether and asepsis? Can you picture the surgeons setting the fractured bones of hundreds of thousands of soldiers and millions of civilians without the use of X-ray? Can you dream of having your kidneys explored for a kidney stone without previously having had an X-ray examination? That would be a nightmare. They knew that pulmonary tuberculosis could be diagnosed by the X-ray and that by a routine examination of the recruits as they were mustered into the service, that tuberculosis could practically have been prevented in the war. Why in the world do you suppose that this was not done? Instead of using the X-ray for the diagnosis of tuberculosis in the army, they based their diagnosis of tuberculosis on the peculiar noises that they heard when they listened for sounds within the chest. They used peculiar tubes that they stuck in their ears. They called them stethoscopes. Can you imagine having your sinuses drained or your mastoids resected without an X-ray examination? Can you imagine people having their bellies opened and being cut up for cancer of the stomach without an X-ray examination? Remember that these were in the days when they tried to cure cancer by cutting it out after it had started rather than preventing it before it started."

This historian of the dim and the distant future will say, "They soon learned that these radiant energies had a profound biologic effect without causing pain, or, in fact, without causing any sensation whatever. It was first noted that the reproductive organs ceased to generate, that is, there was a lack of growth in these particular cells. After this it was observed that other cells of the body began to grow wild when stimulated by this new radiant energy. In other words, this radiant energy caused cancer in a hundred odd victims, who were martyrs to the cause.

"These detrimental effects of the X-ray were largely controlled by protecting the operator, but every now and then a new group of cases would crop up. A spectacular example of the danger of this powerful energy occurred in a group of young girls who worked in applying radium to the dials of watches. Much as you or I would moisten the tip of a lead pencil, they moistened their radium pencils with their tongues, without knowing the silent but deadly energy which they were thus taking into their bodies. They swam, danced, and tried to beat old 'Colonel Bogey' in a game called golf, never dreaming that this new radiant energy on the tip of the tongue was getting in its deadly effects."

The historian of the dim distant future will say, "Strange as it seems, as soon as these people learned that X-ray and radium caused cancer, they began to use it to cure cancer, that is, to destroy or to stunt those cells that had grown wild. These radiant energies which they had come to know by the name of X-ray, radium, infra-red, ultra-violet, and so forth, were but small segments in the cycle of radiant energy that extends to the farthest star in the unexplored universe.

"Therefore, early in the twentieth century, man was far advanced in civilization, if you could call it such. It was then hinted that he might destroy himself and others with these inventions or discoveries, particularly those in the field of radiant energy, the unknown quantity of Roentgen. But it was not until the second World War in the middle of the century that those detrimental and dangerous factors began to be used for the wanton destruction of man."

The medical historian of the twenty-first century will continue to record that it was only recently that there was found in a book published by the New York Academy of Medicine an account relating to an incident that occurred late in the fourth decade. A queer old man, inclined to reminisce and to see visions, was spinning yarns to a group of listeners in a beautiful building that had not yet been destroyed. It must be remembered that at this time in some of the more "kultured" centers of the world many scientific books had already been destroyed, but in the auditorium of this building was assembled a group of isolationists who were complacently repeating the popular slogan, "It can't happen here." This queer old man had been telling them unbelievable things that had happened within the memory of man. He had told them how this unknown quantity, X, had passed through the bodies of victims without causing any discomfort, but that the subjects were rendered sterile on the one hand or developed wildly growing cells of cancer on the other. This audience had been listening for more than an hour and were only mildly interested in his yarns. But when this old man said, "Man-made energy, similar but not identical with that which caused hundreds of victims of cancer, is now passing through each of you," they woke up with a start. Could such a thing be possible? He simply told them to go home and carry out a very simple experiment to prove for themselves that they were constantly exposed to this man-made energy. They were to cut the antennæ of the radio four or five feet from the apparatus, strip the insulation if there was any, tune in on any station, even at the far ends of the earth if they had a short wave set, and listen to political dictators, planning for their own power and glory. Set the amplifier so that the volume of their voices is just barely audible, then moisten thumb and fingers, hold the antennæ, and listen to the booming of their voices. This marked increase in sound, as you hold the ends of the bare antennæ, simply records the man-made energy that is passing through your body twenty-four hours a day from a small segment of the universal circuit of radio energy. These particular waves, which go through our body, even from the top to the bottom of the dial, may not and probably do not have any biologic effect. We do know with certainty, however, that short wave lengths, X-ray and radium, are deadly at short range—though they do not go around the world. And it is not beyond the realm of possibility that other, as yet undiscovered waves of long wave frequency which encircle the globe, may be as deadly as these short waves are at short range.

Mind you, this was in the fourth decade of the twentieth century, before the second World War.

(1)